# Elements of Moral Experience in Clinical Ethics Training and Practice

*Elements of Moral Experience in Clinical Ethics Training and Practice: Sharing Stories with Strangers* is a philosophical and professional memoir of the education, training, and professional development of becoming a clinical ethics consultant. Utilizing a phenomenological and narrative lens, this book offers a fresh and energizing window into the field of healthcare ethics by pairing compelling clinical narratives of what it is like to do clinical ethics consultation with clear reflections and accessible introductions to key philosophical, professional, and humanistic roots for responsible practice. Each chapter contains a firsthand account of a clinical ethics encounter – with vivid detail, verbatim dialogue, and internal monologues that reveal the consultant's reflections throughout the consultation. Following or at times woven into the clinical story, each chapter explores elements of practice by highlighting philosophical, professional, and humanistic resources that connect to and shape meaning in everyday clinical ethics work, drawing from phenomenologically and narratively oriented ethicists (Richard Zaner, Andrea Frolic, Mark Bliton, and Stuart Finder), influential thinkers in adjacent fields (Alfred Schutz, Kurt Wolff, and Pierre Bourdieu), and creative writers and artists (Barry Lopez, Joe Henry, Audre Lorde, Robert M. Pirsig, and Dar Williams). The innovative structure signposts and illustrates distinct elements of clinical ethics experience and practice, inviting the reader to move through the book in different ways, according to their own learning goals, as graduate students, advanced trainees, practicing clinical ethicists, or ethics educators. By focusing on themes identified in the unique instances or experiences of first-hand accounts, or by tracing the philosophical reflections on grounding and orienting texts from the field, readers can access different elements of clinical ethics practice while the book as a whole models a process for considering and interrogating these elements. *Elements of Moral Experience in Clinical Ethics Training and Practice: Sharing Stories With Strangers* invites readers to articulate, reflect on, share, and ultimately learn from their own experiences in clinical ethics consultation.

**Virginia L. Bartlett** is an assistant professor of biomedical sciences and assistant director of the Center for Healthcare Ethics at Cedars-Sinai Medical Center in Los Angeles, CA. She is a past chair of the Clinical Ethics Consultation Affairs committee for the American Society for Bioethics and Humanities.

T0384730

# Elements of Moral Experience in Clinical Ethics Training and Practice

## Sharing Stories with Strangers

**Virginia L. Bartlett**

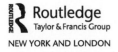
Routledge
Taylor & Francis Group

NEW YORK AND LONDON

Cover image "Transformative Chapter" Duy Huynh ©

First published 2024
by Routledge
605 Third Avenue, New York, NY 10158

and by Routledge
4 Park Square, Milton Park, Abingdon, Oxon, OX14 4RN

*Routledge is an imprint of the Taylor & Francis Group, an informa business*

*British Library Cataloguing-in-Publication Data*
A catalogue record for this book is available from the British Library

*Library of Congress Cataloging-in-Publication Data*
Names: Bartlett, Virginia Latham, author.
Title: Elements of moral experience in clinical ethics training and practice : sharing stories with strangers / Virginia L. Bartlett, PhD.
Description: New York, NY : Routledge, [2024] | Includes bibliographical references and index. | Summary: "Elements of Moral Experience in Clinical Ethics Training and Practice: Sharing Stories with Strangers is a philosophical and professional memoir of the education, training, and professional development of becoming a clinical ethics consultant. Utilizing a phenomenological and narrative lens, this book offers a fresh and energizing window into the field of healthcare ethics by pairing compelling clinical narratives of what it is like to do clinical ethics consultation with clear reflections and accessible introductions to key philosophical, professional, and humanistic roots for responsible practice"-- Provided by publisher.
Identifiers: LCCN 2023026288 (print) | LCCN 2023026289 (ebook) | ISBN 9781032408217 (hardback) | ISBN 9781032408200 (paperback) | ISBN 9781003354864 (ebook)
Subjects: LCSH: Bartlett, Virginia Latham. | Medical ethics--United States--Biography. | Bioethicists--United States--Biography. | Women in medicine--United States--Biography.
Classification: LCC R724 .B333 2024 (print) | LCC R724 (ebook) | DDC 174.2--dc23/eng/20230830
LC record available at https://lccn.loc.gov/2023026288
LC ebook record available at https://lccn.loc.gov/2023026289

ISBN: 978-1-032-40821-7 (hbk)
ISBN: 978-1-032-40820-0 (pbk)
ISBN: 978-1-003-35486-4 (ebk)

DOI: 10.4324/9781003354864

Typeset in Times New Roman
by KnowledgeWorks Global Ltd.

# Contents

# Acknowledgments

For the patients, families, and clinical colleagues too numerous to name, I am grateful beyond measure for your openness and vulnerability, your insights and questions, and the stories you shared with me of your experiences as we shared the experiences in the moral moments of clinical ethics encounters. You have taught me how many ways there are to care for other human beings and to be cared for in return. I daresay most are unaware of how profoundly they have shaped my practice and my professional and personal growth, but I hope that in our moments together they felt heard and felt that they and their stories mattered.

For my predecessors, professional colleagues and peers, I am grateful for the questions and insights, the support and the stories you've shared through conversation, conferencing, and correspondence, in person, by video calls through the pandemic, through your writings both personal and professional. I give special thanks to Dr. Ken Leeds and Dr. Andy Kondrat, my colleagues at Cedars-Sinai for unwavering support, encouragement, and helping me be clear as I can; to Dr. Mindy McGarrah-Sharp, who has offered professional and personal support from graduate school to the present day; and to Dr. Laura Webster, for her professional insights, and caring friendship. I am grateful to Dr. Richard M. Zaner, my teachers' teacher, whose work has so profoundly shaped the field and my own practice, through his creativity and clarity and his deep insistence that stories are at the core of clinical ethics work. And I am grateful to Dr. Leon Morgenstern, of blessed memory, who founded the Bioethics Program at Cedars-Sinai Medical Center, which became the Center for Healthcare Ethics. Leon's deep care for patients and their care providers, and his insistence that I should write every day have inspired me and carried me through the many challenges and iterations of this work. I am grateful to the writers and poets and artists who have infused my life with meaning and wonder through stunning convergences and constellations of discovery. Special thanks to Ms. Dar Williams for permission to quote her beautiful song, "You're Aging Well." Special thanks, also, to Mr. Duy Huynh for allowing me to use his beautiful painting, "Transformative Chapter" as the cover for these transformative chapters.

For my teachers-colleagues-friends, Mark J. Bliton and Stuart G. Finder: thank you. For welcoming my questions and stories, showing me how to pay attention, and demonstrating how to live in and through my own vulnerability in moments of disruption inherent in this work – and in the tricky business of being human. Thank you for showing me what it means to be supported and to support each other – personally and professionally. Thank you for helping me learn to listen *hard* to what all matters in moments of connection with other humans, and thank you for helping me find my voice, especially in the writing of this book. I am grateful for all the stories we share and am looking forward to all those yet to unfold, yet to be told.

For my family – endless thanks to my parents and siblings who have supported me in all I do, and with whom I share stories that shape how I understand and find meaning in the world. My gratitude to my children is boundless as well: they are incandescent beings who make the world shine brighter, and they have taught me how to listen, especially when it's hard, and how to pay attention to both the mundane and the extraordinary. They have made me a better clinician than I could have imagined, and I hope they realize my clinical work has made me a better parent than I would have been otherwise. Sophia, Ellison, and Latham, along with their father, Shane Bartlett, supported this project since it first emerged, even among shifting storylines in our family and our world. All three, along with William and Henry, my bonus children, continue to teach me how to elicit and articulate what matters, how to be flexible and responsive, and how to keep going in the midst of uncertainty, appreciating and loving each other along the way. Finally, I am grateful for the love and support of my partner, Preston Robinson, for the wild serendipity that reconnected us, the deep, old stories that ground us, and for whatever is next as our story together, the story of our family, continues and grows …

# Introduction

"The 'what to do' issue seems the author's and thus is a straw man: Consult. See the parents."
                                                                    – Reviewer # 2, 2012

Once upon a time, early in my career, I wrote about a clinical ethics encounter from the Neonatal Intensive Care Unit. This writing became a paper which explored the consultant's experience of responsibility. My aim was to describe, in an accessible way, what it is like trying to decide what to do among the multiple options available in what are assumed to be the mundane choices and actions that unfold in a clinical consult. The paper was well received at the Annual Meeting for the American Society of Bioethics and Humanities, and so I thought, "Hmmm …, I should turn this into a manuscript." Which I did. The manuscript wasn't accepted (which, of course, is something that happens). More germane to this book was the epiphany gained from reading the reviewer's comments. I was stunned, at least at first, baffled, and then ultimately grateful for the response encapsulated in Reviewer #2's comment above. Why? Although Reviewer #2 gets a bad rap for being the nitpicky pendant, focused on their taken-for-granted method or favorite disciplinary view, the comment made me pay attention to something *I* had taken for granted – in my clinical practice and my writing: *Of course* the "what to do" issue was the author's/consultant's! It is *always* the question for the clinical ethics consultant, isn't it? *Isn't it?*

It turns out not, and so Reviewer #2's comment over a decade ago clarified what has become a set of questions, threaded together at the core of my own practice: What is it like to actually *do* clinical ethics work? How do we practice responsibly as individuals? And how do we do this work together as part of a community, a field? These questions shape my daily practice and have informed much of my scholarship. Over time, they became the motivating concerns for writing this book, which answers each question with its subtitle: *Sharing Stories with Strangers*. What is it like to actually do clinical ethics work? A lot like sharing stories with strangers. How do we do this work responsibly as individuals? We can answer that question only if we are responsible in sharing stories with strangers. And how do we do this work together as part of a community and field? You guessed it! Through sharing stories with strangers. And exploring the depths and layers, the variations and nuances in what it means to share stories with strangers gets to the heart of clinical ethics work.

Clinical ethics consultation includes an array of communicative practices oriented and organized by careful inquiry into the moral and ethical concerns that arise in healthcare settings, and therefore involves having conversations with the people whose concerns these actually are, including patients, families, and clinicians. As clinical ethics consultants, we elicit and listen to and learn from the stories that patients, family members, and clinicians share in consultation conversations. The focus is on the specificity of *this* encounter, with *these* people facing questions and uncertainties

DOI: 10.4324/9781003354864-1

in *their* own particular circumstances. We often retell *those* encounters in case reports, conference papers, or publications, as part of our professional engagement and development, sharing others' stories as examples of themes or concerns that, while unique to them, are also common or familiar across other healthcare contexts and practice settings. The communicative nature of clinical ethics work spans the specificity and depth of conversations in consultation encounters to the scope and reach of discussions about themes, issues, and topics that generate requests for clinical ethics consultation.

And yet, as individuals and a field, we are less likely to communicate and share stories about *our experiences as clinical ethics consultants*. In the legitimating forums of presentation and publication, an ethics consultants' stories about *their* own experiences often are disregarded as too individual and idiosyncratic, as not contributing to what are claimed as the *real* ethics issues. Given the increasingly prominent models in this field that make claims for authoritative expertise, standardized procedural approaches, and exam-certified legitimacy, clinical ethics encounters – the moral moments *we* experience – are expected to get neutralized and anonymized, tamed and flattened into "case studies" or "examples" for "kinds" of consults.[1] The consultants' experiences are excluded and excised from the tale, seemingly unwelcome. Not only does this exclusion serve to create doubt that our personal experiences and insights are somehow considered as legitimate sources of understanding, it serves to alienate diverse forms of moral practice across different communal contexts.

The guide for this book, the invitation to you, dear reader, is that *stories* do not have to be generalized and they can serve a different purpose in our practices. Stories are personal. Interpersonal. Intersubjective. Stories convey values and moral insight in those ways we embody and model our responsibilities when telling them – and when listening to and receiving them. Stories shared among clinical ethics consultants can create communities of understanding about this work, connected by pathways through provinces of meaning. Even when we discover meanings that don't always fit into predetermined frameworks in one or another view about "ethics," our stories can illuminate elements of actual practice and invite reflection on what may be common among our unique experiences.

After all, stories of particular consultants' practices *do* emerge and they circulate in conversation, shared within our communities of practice. Our stories come out in the conversations *after* presentations at a conference; in discussions around the coffee station or across the bar or over the dinner table with peers from other institutions; colleagues and friends from other places and times. These are the stories that make people wince with remembrance of their own moments; or nod slowly, listening carefully to the strange newness; or bust out an awkward guffaw of recognition and fellow feeling from the absurdities that pepper clinical experience. These are the stories we tell each other and ourselves, about the work we do and how and why.

In my tradition, practice as a clinical ethics consultant means taking seriously the moral dimensions unfolding in a particular encounter, and part of developing a responsible practice is engagement *with the specifics of one's particular practice*, as well as with insights from the broader field and how colleagues and peers engage with their practice. Like all stories, our clinical experiences require tellings-and-listenings for their meanings to emerge in the spaces among speakers and audience, or writers and readers. Stories shape our practices, and our understandings of this work we do together.

So, inspired both by the clinical ethics encounters that stay with me *as stories* and by comments like the one that stuck with me from Reviewer #2, much of my professional engagement has explored the question of "what to do" or "what we do" as a live and lively concern, rather than as already answered. Specifically, over the years I've wound up writing my experiences as stories as a way of trying to get clear about what just happened and what all mattered in each encounter or experience. As the collection of recollections has grown, I've realized that all of them illustrate what I have grown to think of as elements of or facets of responsibility in doing clinical ethics work, which together form what Richard M. Zaner called "a general method."[2] Over time, through writing these stories and reflections on my experience as the clinical ethics consultant, I have engaged what other thinkers in the field have thought about these elements of practice, and explored other, additional resources – philosophical, literary, creative arts – seeking perspectives that might help me think about these elements of clinical ethics.

With what I have learned is the not insignificant amount of time required to coax these things into view, those efforts were likewise shaped into this book, *The Elements of Moral Experience in Clinical Ethics Training and Practice: Sharing Stories with Strangers,* a bricolage structured to invite reflection on the stories we share and the elements of practice they reveal. Each chapter includes one or more stories of a clinical ethics encounter that illustrate a specific element of practice, followed by reflections to draw from an array of resources, seeking from a cacophony of voices. Drawn from stories and songs as well as philosophy, sociology, anthropology, and clinical ethics literature, these voices offer insights and explanations that help to find ways to understand meaning in clinical encounters. The aim in this structure is to enable the reader to engage in ways that best suit their needs: each story can be read on its own, as can the reflections. Or each chapter can be engaged as a whole, or each of the three parts – with two chapters each – could be read to focus on specific elements: Discovery, Learning, or Experience. Or the reader could read from start to finish, following the arc of the book, though with the caveat that everything circles back around to the questions with which we began: What is it like to actually *do* clinical ethics work? How do we practice responsibly as individuals? And how do we do this work together as part of a community, a field? The brief outline that follows might serve as a guide for the perplexed.

## Elements of Clinical Ethics Practice

Part I: Elements of Discovery focuses on the experience of *unknowing* in clinical ethics work, experiences elicited through disruption and strangeness. These are worked through by the careful focusing of attention and the experiences of surrender-and-catch, which can be engaged and enacted as part of practice and method in clinical ethics work.

Chapter 1, "Seminar in Strangeness" introduces the unavoidable, inherent disruption and *strangeness* of clinical ethics work. "Observations I," "Stairwell Stories I," and "Observations II" illustrate the disconcerting experiences of discovering that clinical ethics – and clinical philosophy – was different than imagined: more interpersonal, reflective, and requiring vulnerability for communication and understanding. Chapter 1 uses Alfred Schutz's 1944 essay "The Stranger"[3] to explore the experiences of disruption, uncertainty, and navigating meaning-making constituent of clinical ethics work – and models the focus, reflection, and careful attention that became a method of doing clinical philosophy outside the classroom.

Chapter 2, "Clinical Attention as Surrender-and-Catch," explores attention as an element in clinical ethics work: the attention that is deliberately directed and the attention that is elicited by disruptive occasions or encounters. After the story, "Mr. Jones and Me," the chapter alternates between journal excerpts from my first clinical rotations in the Medical Intensive Care Unit (MICU), and reflection on sociologist Kurt Wolff's generative and wondrously peculiar book, *Surrender and Catch: Experience and Inquiry Today.*[4] These reflections provide clinical and practical frames for understanding – particularly the unexpected surrender-and-catch, and more deliberate process of surrender-to: both ever-present possibilities in clinical ethics work.

Part I ends with an "Interlude I: Methods of Unknowing: Disruption and Attention" to explore disruption/strangeness and surrender-and-catch together as a kind of *method* of unknowing and hence openness to discovery. The inevitable unknowing and the humbling acceptance that neither the Stranger's careful approach nor the deliberate attention of the surrender-to may be sufficient for understanding and action serve as an access point to deliberate inquiry, and ongoing learning, as part of responsible practice.

Part II: Elements of Learning focuses on practices of self-reflection and self-education, as these occur with others, through practices of affiliation and attunement. Chapter 3, "Self-Reflection and Self-Education in Clinical Ethics" explores the need to recognize rigor in self-reflection as a crucial component of method in clinical ethics work, illustrated through a clinical encounter from my training in the Neonatal Intensive Care Unit (NICU).[5] The story, "Unexpected Invitations," unfolds through journal excerpts from my months in the NICU and is framed by anthropologist and clinical ethicist Andrea Frolic's call for embodied self-reflection in clinical ethics work[6] and philosopher Harald Ofstad's reminder – from over 40 years ago – that self-reflection, as a necessary part of moral education, is not a merely solitary activity.[7]

Chapter 4, "Affiliation and Attunement: Extra-ordinary Discourse" is the longest and most central chapter for the book. This chapter dives into the details of such interpersonal connection in clinical ethics by explicating two key elements: attunement and affiliation. These elements are illustrated by "Me and the MOMS," a story of an encounter with a pregnant woman and her partner considering experimental prenatal surgery for their fetus with spina bifida. The interpersonal and moral features are examined through the sociological and clinical-philosophical lenses of Pierre Bourdieu, Richard M. Zaner, and Mark J. Bliton.[8] The encounter – and the philosophical reflections that followed – serve as a pivot point and key recognition of clinical ethics as a moral activity and extraordinary discourse.

Part II: Elements of Learning ends with "Interlude II: Learning with Others: Vulnerability and Sharing Stories," which reviews how elements of self-reflection and self-education, along with affiliation and attunement are constituent and necessary for responsible clinical ethics practice. Drawing from the example of *Peer Review, Peer Education, and Modeling in the Practice of Clinical Ethics Consultation: The Zadeh Project*, Stuart Finder and Mark Bliton's edited volume on peer learning,[9] Interlude II helps frame the questions that shape the final third of the book: how do we talk about or share, find meaning in, and give accounts of our own moral moments and encounters with others? What do we do if we recognize the vulnerability of such moments, and how do we respond when the encounter exposes our own affiliations, commitments, or unacknowledged biases? When our experiences put *us* into question?

Part III: Elements of Experience thus considers experiences of clinical ethics work through the ethics consultant's vulnerability – and through the practice of telling our own stories of our own experiences. Chapter 5, "Constituent Vulnerability, Constituent Responsibility" explores vulnerability as an unavoidable, inherent element of responsibility in clinical ethics practice. It begins with "We Are Power" and "Afterwards/After Words," stories of a wrenching clinical encounter with struggling clinicians and a grieving family that illustrate the multiple forms of and expressions of vulnerability that clinical ethics consultants experience. This chapter draws philosophical insights from Barry Hoffmaster's reflections in "What Does Vulnerability Mean?"[10]; Herbert Spiegelberg about responsibility in "Ethics for Fellows in the Fate of Existence"[11]; and from Richard M. Zaner's "Power and Hope in the Clinical Encounter: a Meditation on Vulnerability."[12]

Finally, Chapter 6, "Clinical Storytelling and Fragments of Experience" wrestles with the challenge of clinical ethics consultants sharing our own moral experiences and exploring their meanings with others. This element in clinical ethics practice emerges in "Later That Same Day: The "Cameron Story"" the story of a moment where I nearly fainted mid-consult, in the room with a patient requesting a legally prescribed lethal medication to end her life via medical aid-in-dying. The reflections explore the rigors of telling and making sense of that disruption, exposure, shame, and uncertainty that shuddered and rippled like shockwaves out from that moment. The reflections on this encounter emerge as fragments, possibly the most fitting genre for brief reflections on the limits of clinical storytelling and narrative approaches to ethics, and to do this I draw from reflective resources in literature, song, and creative arts. These diverse genres are intended highlight modes of imaginative engagement that support sharing and understanding, accounting for the wild serendipity and anarchy of voices in human experiences, especially in clinical encounters.

The work doesn't end, although the book does, concluding with "Sharing Stories with Strangers: Continuing When There is No Ending": exploring ideas regarding un-get-around-able orientations and core elements necessary for responsible practice in clinical ethics work. They also reflect what I see as the necessity for stories and shared reflection in clinical ethics work, particularly the need to recognize these practices of discovering and excavating *meaning* as necessary to illustrate the richly layered, iterative, and ongoing experiences *that are the work*.

### Keep Us in Song: Clinical Ethics, Phenomenology, and Sharing Stories with Strangers

The stories that follow are offered as examples of the everyday, the mundane phenomenon of clinical ethics work – both the experiences of the clinical moments as well as the discernable moral insights gathered by reflecting and learning from them (a process without strict beginning or end, I'll note). They offer access to the even stranger phenomenon of attempting to capture these stories on a page and share them with others – with readers-as-strangers. I offer my stories of my experiences in clinical ethics work, with the invitation for others to read, to consider, to ask, probe, argue, as a spur for reflection on *their* access to and experience with or understandings of the phenomenon of clinical ethics consultation. These stories of mine are offered humbly and proudly.

Humbly in the knowledge that as a phenomenological work, it is partial and particular and as a collection of stories or memoir, it struggles in the bounds of the genre, not designed to offer any steps or advice one might expect in an account of professional development. These stories have no aphorism at the end, not single moral or meaning – even if they *are* about moral elements of clinical ethics practice. People will find much to dispute and challenge and question – and that is by design.

It is also offered proudly, for many of the same reasons, in keeping with the moral dialogue we so desperately need. People will find much to consider and question and dispute and chew on – good! Whether the response is "What nonsense!" or "I had that *same experience!*" or "That essay she references is old news" or "I don't even know who that thinker is ..." May your conversations be fruitful – with yourself and your peers, with your trainees and mentors. May you share your stories with strangers and accept theirs in return, learning from each other what it is like to do this work, alone and together.

### Notes

1  Rasmussen, Lisa (2018). Standardizing the Case Narrative. In Stuart G. Finder and Mark J. Bliton (eds.), *Peer Review, Peer Education, and Modeling in the Practice of Clinical Ethics Consultation: The Zadeh Project*. Cham, Switzerland: Springer Verlag. pp. 151–160.
2  Zaner, Richard M. (1988) *Ethics and the Clinical Encounter*. Englewood Cliffs, NJ: Prentice Hall.
3  Schutz, Alfred (1944). The Stranger: An Essay in Social Psychology. *American Journal of Sociology* 49 (6):499–507.
4  Wolff, Kurt H. (1976). Surrender and Catch: Experience and Inquiry Today. In *Boston Studies in the Philosophy and History of Science*, vol. 51. Dordrecht: Springer.
5  N.b. This is *not* the story that Reviewer #2 found unsatisfactory.
6  Frolic, Andrea (2011). Who are we when we are doing what we are doing? The case for mindful embodiment in ethics case consultation. *Bioethics* 25 (7):370–382.

7 Ofstad, Harald (1974). Education versus growth in moral development. *The Monist* 58 (4):581–599.
8 Bourdieu, Pierre (1999). Understanding. In Pierre Bourdieu (ed.), *The Weight of the World: Social Suffering in Contemporary Society*. Cambridge, UK: Polity Press. pp. 607–626. Bliton, Mark J. (2008). Maternal-Fetal Surgery and the 'Profoundest Question in Ethics'. In Paul J. Ford and Denise M. Dudzinski (eds.), *Complex Ethics Consultations: Cases That Haunt Us*. Cambridge, UK: Cambridge University Press. pp. 36–42. See also fn 2, fn 4 above.
9 Finder, Stuart G. and Bliton, Mark J. (eds.) (2018). *Peer Review, Peer Education, and Modeling in the Practice of Clinical Ethics Consultation: The Zadeh Project*. Cham, Switzerland: Springer Verlag.
10 Hoffmaster, Barry (2006). What does vulnerability mean? *Hastings Center Report* 36(2):38–45.
11 Spiegelberg, H. (1986). Ethics for Fellows in the Fate of Existence. In *Steppingstones Toward an Ethics for Fellow Existers*: Essays 1944–1983. Springer. pp. 199–218.
12 Zaner, Richard M. (2000). Power and hope in the clinical encounter: A meditation on vulnerability. *Medicine, Health Care and Philosophy* 3 (3):263–273.

## Bibliography

Bliton, Mark J. and Finder, Stuart G. (2018). The Zadeh Project – A Frame for Understanding the Generative Ideas, Formation, and Design. In Stuart G. Finder and Mark J. Bliton (eds.), *Peer Review, Peer Education, and Modeling in the Practice of Clinical Ethics Consultation: The Zadeh Project*. Cham, Switzerland: Springer Verlag. pp. 1–18.

Bourdieu, Pierre (1999). Understanding. In Pierre Bourdieu (eds.), *The Weight of the World: Social Suffering in Contemporary Society*. Cambridge, UK: Polity Press. pp. 607–626.

Finder, Stuart G. and Bliton, Mark J. (eds.) ( 2018). *Peer Review, Peer Education, and Modeling in the Practice of Clinical Ethics Consultation: The Zadeh Project*. Springer Verlag.

Frolic, Andrea (2011). Who are we when we are doing what we are doing? The case for mindful embodiment in ethics case consultation. *Bioethics* 25 (7):370–382.

Hoffmaster, Barry (2006). What does vulnerability mean? *Hastings Center Report* 36 (2):38–45.

Ofstad, Harald (1974). Education versus growth in moral development. *The Monist* 58 (4):581–599.

Rasmussen, Lisa (2018). Standardizing the Case Narrative. In Stuart G. Finder and Mark J. Bliton (eds.), *Peer Review, Peer Education, and Modeling in the Practice of Clinical Ethics Consultation: The Zadeh Project*. Cham, Switzerland: Springer Verlag. pp. 151–160.

Schutz, Alfred (1944). The Stranger: An Essay in Social Psychology. *American Journal of Sociology* 49 (6):499–507.

Spiegelberg, Herbert (1986). Ethics for Fellows in the Fate of Existence. In *Steppingstones Toward an Ethics for Fellow Existers: Essays 1944–1983*. Springer. pp. 199–218.

Wolff, Kurt H. (1976). Surrender and Catch: Experience and Inquiry Today. In Boston Studies in the Philosophy and History of Science, vol. 51. Dordrecht: Springer.

Zaner, Richard M. (1988). *Ethics and the Clinical Encounter*. Englewood Cliffs, NJ: Prentice Hall.

Zaner, Richard M. (2000). Power and hope in the clinical encounter: A meditation on vulnerability. *Medicine, Health Care and Philosophy* 3 (3):263–273.

# Part I
# Elements of Discovery

# 1  Seminar in Strangeness

**Observations I: Seminar in Clinical Philosophy, October 2003**

The tears erupted silently and fell hot on the page, smudging the ink on the paper where I had been taking notes. They were tears of frustration, I knew. It wasn't sadness or even anger, necessarily. More like furious internal recriminations over my inability to say clearly what I wanted to say, plus an astonishing resentment that simmered toward those four wide open eyes, staring expectantly from behind two pair of glasses – one professor on either side of the table. Finder and Bliton didn't seem to get it, *wouldn't* get it, didn't care how ridiculous I felt in my tongue-tied distress.

My fellow classmates were a three-part study in awkwardness, a triptych of discomfort. Kyle's eyes ping-ponged from me to the professors, Stuart Finder and Mark Bliton; Cherita carefully examined her pen-tip; Joe – who had taken the Seminar before, looked at me sideways, down the table, earnest sympathy and a clearly too-optimistic smile of encouragement hovering. My momentary exasperation at their silence – leaving me floundering for words – was now compounded by the embarrassment of capping my ineffectual engagement with tears. They all just waited: awkwardly or encouragingly, or simply curiously, in the case of the professors. They just waited and watched, with their glasses and beards and wide, open eyes: Finder with his head tilted slightly, like a robin watching the meandering of a pill bug, Bliton tugging absently at the ends of his Vandyke. I wondered if this was some sort of philosophical hazing – with the two of them acting the stereotype to match the phenotype. What on earth did they expect me to do or say now? Why didn't they have the courtesy to move on, to let me contain myself? To ask someone else a question or otherwise fill in that dreadful, wretched silence? Not quite silence, I thought, as I sniffed and cleared my throat, too loudly for the moment. I looked down at my smudged notes.

"This question – what the author has written here – raises some real, as in actual, real for us – the readers – questions. As readers, as people, these are real *live* questions, as William James would say, that are deeply challenging."

Thank God, finally, I thought, at last daring to lift my glasses and wipe my eyes, as everyone's heads swiveled toward Bliton's measured voice.

"Virginia, can you help us understand what this raised for you? It was clearly having an effect, and that seems like it might be helpful to probe a bit and try to understand what is at stake … in that effect, in your response …"

They weren't going to let it go. I couldn't believe it. I glared at Bliton, I blinked once, willing away the sharp, hot pressure of more tears and I took a breath. My words came out clipped, precise,

DOI: 10.4324/9781003354864-3

and slow, as I tried to answer his question, tried to get back to what had so completely disrupted me in the minutes-that-lasted-hours before my tears started. I held onto the printed text in front of me and stabbed my finger to the passage I'd highlighted the night before, avoiding the eyes now back on me, grounding myself by pointing to the point that seemed so crucial. "What I was *trying* to say is that in the author's claim, here, it seems clear she means to highlight …"

## Stairwell Stories I: Vanderbilt University Medical Center, Main Hospital Lobby

The glint of challenge in his eyes met the clenched jaw of my determination, hidden behind my cheerful smile.

"I don't mind taking the stairs," I said.

"The ICU is the seventh floor, are you sure?" Stuart was giving me the out.

"Totally fine," I lied.

This moment – eight seconds, maybe ten, tops – turned out to have been my first failure in my clinical ethics training, though by no means would it be the last. The moment was a failure of listening and of integrity, but in both, an opportunity for learning.

It was a failure of hearing and understanding. I didn't hear my teacher's question about stairs versus elevator as a real question – a live Jamesian option. I heard it as a test, a command, or, perhaps more gently, an unspoken instruction, a push toward a preferred answered. Stuart was asking about my preference or choice, and I misunderstood it as an insinuation about what he expected to see happen, or how he thought I should answer. I started climbing seven flights of stairs because I thought I was being tested. I'd gotten this far in my life by being able to get the right answer on tests, and in the beginning, I approached my clinical ethics training with the same orientation.

The moment was a failure of integrity as well. It was my first day of "real" clinical ethics training, my first day of "clinical exposure": ethics observations – rounding in the Medical Intensive Care Unit. I was so focused on meeting expectations (imagined, projected, and assumed) that I lied. I did not want to climb the stairs. I would not have wanted to climb them under most circumstances, but especially not that day, after I had spent almost fourteen hours of the previous day as a patient in the emergency department of that same hospital I was now entering as an observer.

\*\*\*

I had gone into the Emergency Room after a sleepless Saturday night with worsening pain in my abdomen and back, radiating from my left side. They worked me up (slowly if not quite thoroughly) and sent me home on Sunday evening with a diagnosis of a urinary tract infection, a prescription for antibiotics and pain medicine, and advice to drink cranberry juice and water. This was also a failure, I would come to discover, but at the time I was glad to go home and sleep if I could.

I could not sleep, or at least not well. So, at seven o'clock Monday morning, in a hallway off the lobby of the hospital, I was tired and knew I looked it, looking at Stuart's enquiring face. I felt like roadkill, and my side alternated between a dull ache and prickling spikes of agony. Scaling seven sets of steps was the last thing I wanted to do, but I really wanted to start my "real" ethics training. In that eagerness – and out of my own unarticulated assumptions about what was at expected and at stake – I ignored my own needs and experiences.

We started up the stairs.

\*\*\*

Stuart didn't say anything as we rounded the landing between the fourth and fifth floors, but he looked back while I paused to catch my breath. He paused, his gaze curious. It invited explanation.

I nodded and resumed the stairs, stumbling, short of breath, through the story of the emergency department visit. Stuart slowed his pace to match mine, moving deliberately up each riser, and I found myself responding to his questions with more detail, revealing more emotion and reflection than I intended. As we approached the sixth floor, he offered the elevator again, but at this point, I resolved to power through the path I had chosen. He shrugged, just slightly, and we kept on.

In that accepting shrug, I recognized my failures of the whole moment. My failure to hear his questions as real – not *pro forma*. My failure to honor my experience with integrity, to understand what was at stake for myself and others. I realized that Stuart truly hadn't wanted to continue in one way over the other, but he was going to let me go on however I needed to go on. He was giving me the space to be responsible for my choices – and would walk with me through the consequences. A stunning lesson, a blueprint for the rest of my clinical ethics training and practice.

Or, put another way, in those brief conversations and those eternal minutes trudging up the stairs, Stuart modeled key elements of clinical ethics practice that I would continue to encounter, discover, and rediscover in every other clinical environment from that moment forward. A masterclass, in a flash. An opportunity for learning in a moment, the kind of learning I continue to explore, to practice, to articulate and share with others, and maybe even to understand. Even if just for a moment, only in a moment.

## Observations II: Seminar in Clinical Philosophy, October 2009

They let me talk, uninterrupted. Their eyes were pinned to my face while I looked at the table, or the ceiling. I was looking back into my memory – trying to reclaim and recount what I saw, what I said and heard. I searched for their eyes when something came out clearly – did they hear it? Did they recognize the truth of what I meant to say, even if it didn't come out quite perfectly? Their eyes and attention were there, waiting, every time I looked up to find it. Mindy, Dan, Kyle – my fellow students – along with Jan van Eys, an emeritus professor, and Mark Bliton, my teacher and mentor. The current iteration of Seminar, gathered around the blandly corporate conference table at the Center for Biomedical Ethics and Society. This conference room was as sunny as the old one in Oxford House, but with plate glass windows and clean lines instead of the dusty bookshelves and just-shy-of-overgrown plants. The space didn't matter so much, except that it was an enclosed one, hushed and protected, while I tried to get out what I had gone through.

I had returned the day before from a three-day road trip from Nashville up to my folks' place in East Tennessee. I had taken Sophia, age seven months, with me. She was to stay with my mother and grandmother while I drove over the mountains to North Carolina for my third research interview for my dissertation.

I told my colleagues – my classmates and teachers – how the four-hour trip took over six, as I kept stopping so I could nurse or otherwise try to soothe my wailing banshee of a baby. Mindy nodded with sympathy as I wryly described the decision, after the third stop, to just keep driving and how Sophia and I sobbed in two-part harmony for the last exhausting hour. Mark chuckled as I explained how guilty I felt for being happy that I was able to leave the baby with my mom and drive by myself to my interviewee's house, even though it was pouring rain and the mountain roads were dangerously coated in pea-soup fog. The story became less amusing, and the telling and listening both became more intense as I began to talk of my arrival at the house of the woman to whom I had given the pseudonym of "Carin Miller."

Haltingly, quietly, I tried to explain how it felt "off" and askew from the beginning: the sense of danger – that I was a danger – to this woman, who had agreed to be interviewed about her experiences with prenatal surgery for spina bifida and ethics consultation. How the woman who had invited me to their home so enthusiastically during our initial phone call a week ago appeared to have closed down before she opened the door. How the welcome and introductions to her husband and her daughter, the child with spina bifida, were polite and brittle, and how the answers to my questions, as we sat around her dining room table, were so contained and constrained as to be conversational deadends. My throat caught as I tried to describe Carin's stricken eyes, how the film of tears kept them bright throughout the interview; how those eyes stared at me intently as I asked my questions, but they flitted between her husband, her daughter, and the floor when she answered. How George, her husband, appeared overly cheerful and deliberately vague: "Oh, we don't really think about that," "Oh, it was so long ago, I'm not really sure." I looked at Mark as I explained that every question got harder to ask, as Carin's posture visibly tightened, as if she were bracing herself for something – for the question that would unravel all of her control, all of her mastery of emotion and memory and experience. Dan, the sociologist, nodded a quick, short nod as I described my growing self-doubt about the purpose of these questions and whether I should keep asking. Does my project, my curiosity, my need to learn outweigh her obvious distress, the sense that I was causing harm by asking her about this experience in her life? Was I projecting my own distress as I listened to their stories of their traumatic delivery and subsequent diagnoses? Hearing them describe their upended lives, both made richer and completely dismantled by their longed-for child, who is different than the child they imagined in their longing? Was it my guilt when I thought about my healthy, lively baby that caused the growing sense of voyeurism as they shut down each question so completely with the barest of responses? It had all mattered – every moment, every word – and none of my preparation had prepared me for their barnacled grief, sharp below the water line of our conversation.

Even as I asked them the next question on my thoroughly researched and thoughtfully constructed interview guide, my eyes sank with the weight of the questions I asked myself, silently, in my head. Should I be responsible to the project and keep going with the questions? Am I responsible for calling a halt, for wrapping it up when I see, or imagine I see, how awful this is for her? Or is she responsible for voicing her distress if it's too much, since she agreed to talk with me? And if it's me, should I be explicit and deliberate, giving her the chance to carry on if she wants to and can? Or do I exit as gracefully, as indirectly as possible, trying not to compound the harm of making her feel bad about her lack of engagement, such a short conversation? What will be least harmful as this interview stretches out, from discomfort into dismay, distress, disaster?

Jan and Mindy exchanged glances as I tried to explain the passage of time: how I knew on one level that this interview was shorter than the others I had conducted, shorter than the interview guide should have allowed, and yet it felt like the afternoon had gone on all day. It seemed as though Carin and George and I couldn't get out of the moment.

As I looked around the shining, dark cherry table at the faces of my friends and mentors, I recognized that I was still in the moment. I was still wide open and vulnerable and, uncertain, wracked by the sense of connection, of affiliation, with these strangers who let me into their home for a brief hour. And I recognized with wonder and relief that rather than getting me out of it, *these* not-quite-strangers, my Seminar colleagues, were joining me in it, wrapping me in *their* affiliation, their willingness, and their practiced efforts to understand.

Their questions were careful and gentle, pointed and probing. Details about where Carin and George and I sat in relation to each other and about what their daughter was doing; reflective questions asking if I knew what I was thinking at this moment or that, if I could recall how I had phrased a particular query, or what I saw in Carin's voice, face, words that made me think she was overwhelmed and wonder if I should stop. Had I considered an alternative interpretation of Carin and George's poor memory? Remember when we read Bourdieu on *Understanding* and the connection and investment of the interviewer? Could I imagine what might have made the interview different? My colleagues imagined with me, listening closely, attending to and responding to what I said, and helping me excavate what was *Unsaid*. They helped me speak what I hadn't realized I was thinking and helped me identify and account for the nuances of my experience. Sitting around the Seminar table, noting the care with which my colleagues joined me in trying to understand my experiences, I started understanding some of what I was *still* experiencing – layers and facets that I could not access from my deep involvement, from the isolation and particularity of my encounter. And when I felt the tears – of sadness for this family into whose life I intruded – I didn't rush to wipe them away, to hide the overwhelm, to pretend I was not affected by this deeply personal, deeply moral encounter with another. I took a long, slow breath, grateful for the care, I can even say the *love*, with which my colleagues supported this experience of learning together.

### The Clinical Part of Clinical Ethics or, Strangeness in the Seminar in Clinical Philosophy

Seminar was the beginning of my becoming a clinical ethics consultant because Seminar was the beginning of my learning how to be a Stranger. This first requires some elaboration and clarification about why learning how to become a Stranger has something to do with Clinical Ethics, and an explanation of about why and how a Seminar in Clinical Philosophy helped me learn how to be a Stranger.

Many people conflate clinical ethics with bioethics as applied ethics coming from academic, philosophical study of ethics. I certainly had that impression when I started my master's program. From what I had read as an undergraduate and my first brief forays into the literature around medical ethics/healthcare ethics/bioethics as a graduate student, I thought I was going to learn about theories and frameworks. I thought I would learn how to apply them to dilemmas in medical or healthcare settings and be able to identify the "right" thing to do or the "right choice" from a neutral, rational "ethics" perspective. I thought of ethics as a thing to be learned – information to be acquired and processed, used and mastered. I hadn't even heard of "clinical ethics" as a particular field or practice – but the description of a "Seminar in Clinical Philosophy" cross-listed in the Divinity School course catalog was intriguing. I enrolled, eager and ready to learn and get started on the "real" bioethics work. Though Seminar was unique to Vanderbilt's Center for Clinical and Research Ethics, I have learned over the years from conversations with others in our field about similar experiences with a learning cohort, course, or community where they learned how to engage and reflect on practice as they developed their practice. I've also learned that not everyone has had such experiences in formal educational or training sessions, although some have created or encountered their own – and these unique but similar or parallel experiences can be a starting point for conversation within the field about our training – and how we learn to engage with our ongoing practices of learning.

Seminar started at the Center as a set of independent readings and emerging questions in the fall of 1993, which was formalized into a course with a structured syllabus in the fall of 1994. It had the typical appearance of a seminar – the usual trappings: set meeting times, a room with a conference table, taking attendance, agreed-upon readings. The readings were impressive: practical pieces and theoretical pieces; clinical pieces – medical and nursing journal articles, ethics consultation case reports; social sciences; literature and poetry. All aimed at generating conversation about what mattered in caring about and in caring for other human beings what was *worthwhile*.

The readings, however, were not the focus. They were the hook, the door: the invitation to the actual *work* of Seminar. The work of Seminar was listening and talking and discovering with these fellow strangers what each other thought and understood, focusing on questions arising in clinical contexts. The discipline of Seminar was radically questioning – an iterative practice of giving an account of one's thinking, one's position, one's questions, one's biases and commitments, a practice of probing, or, as is detailed in the starting assumption on the very first Seminar syllabus:

> This is a seminar in clinical philosophy. As such, while we recognize that each participant – including ourselves – enters into the seminar with some commitment or another ..., we expect participants to have a willingness to put into question their own commitments as we all pursue what's at stake in the pursuit of well-being.
>
> (Syllabus, Spring 1993)

Rather than setting aside or ignoring those commitments in favor of the "ethics issues," as if those were some isolated subject matter, Seminar practice insisted that our values and commitments necessarily shaped how we approached and understood any subject or question, such that our understanding became an object of study and understanding as much as the prompting texts.

As "Observations I" and "Observations II," along with the "Stairwell Stories," illustrate, Seminar was not what I had expected from previous seminars in graduate school, nor were the challenges encountered through my clinical ethics observations in the Medical Intensive Care Unit what I had imagined. Seminar insisted that "ethics issues" and "moral quandaries" didn't exist in some free-floating form, to be identified "out there," to be analyzed into submission and applied universally. I had not expected the immediacy and intensity of realizing that the fact I was there in the first place was an ethical issue, a moral encounter. In Seminar and even in my approach to that first day in a clinical setting, I was at stake, and had to be responsible for myself: my thoughts and my questions, my actions, my inactions. My teachers, Mark Bliton and Stuart Finder, cared about how we read the texts, how we thought about the issues raised, and how we engaged with and learned from each other. We were *doing* clinical ethics work by exploring issues that arise in clinical settings – even when we were sitting around a conference room table. The ethical perspectives included those we carried with us, which meant we had to be clear about them and accountable for them – even when we didn't even recognize them until others pointed out what we took for granted. The realization that I could not be a bystander – that I was going to be in question myself – was part of the deep disruption and strangeness of Seminar.

Over time, the idea became clearer that clinical ethics work, as a practice, was infinitely more complex and stranger than the "casebooks" and theoretical works showed. Although it took me years to truly absorb and accept the idea of clinical ethics as a moral activity rather than an academic exercise, eventually I recognized that clinical ethics was not just mediating disputes between patients and physicians or following a set of rules or analytic structures. Seminar made clear that the ethics consultant, individually, even if part of a team, was responsible for helping people navigate their unique experiences of illness or injury, caring for or being cared for by others, and figuring out what's going on, what all matters, and how they might go forward in their own disruption and in the aftermaths of choices. More striking in that realization, perhaps, was the recognition that the ethics consultant was not protected from the disruption of others and was not immune from their own experience of disruption: uncertainty, upheaval, and unknowing. The readings and conversations in Seminar required consideration of the human, the moral elements of clinical ethics work – and the experience of disruption as a constituent element of clinical ethics work. The question for practice thus emerged: how do we, as ethics consultants, recognize, live in, and learn from the unchosen disruptions in the context of healthcare and healing – those of others and when we encounter our own?

In Seminar and in my early clinical exposures, I struggled with and against the idea of disruption as anything but a negative. Uncertainty and unknowing, disruption and disequilibrium seemed like experiences to be avoided if possible and ameliorated if not. However, my experiences – in Seminar and ICU – made clear that clinical ethics required eliciting, clarifying, and communicating about the concerns and values at stake for the patients, families, and clinicians involved at moments when *they* are disrupted and unsettled. To engage with others in their disruption and their experiences of uncertainty meant I had to get comfortable with my own discomfort, and my own uncertainties and strangeness. Hence, the idea of the Stranger is one I found helpful as a frame for the strangeness and disruption of Seminar and of clinical ethics work.

### Encountering the Stranger with Alfred Schutz

The idea of the Stranger pops up periodically as a motif in clinical ethics. Richard Zaner explores the concept, as do Larry Churchill,[1] David Barnard,[2] Edward Tiraykian,[3] and George Agich.[4] Each has used the idea to address different concerns regarding practice, role, educational approaches, and other topics in bioethics and clinical ethics.

A core understanding of this concept and its relevance to the *experience* of clinical ethics consultants, and as an *orientation and method* for practice in clinical ethics consultation, comes from one of the philosophers whose work I encountered for the first time in Seminar: Alfred Schutz. Widely respected and influential as a scholar and a teacher, Schutz is perhaps an underrecognized contributor to clinical ethics work, so a brief review of his work, especially his 1944 essay "The Stranger: An Essay in Social Psychology"[5] will help put the strangeness of clinical ethics in context.

### The Strange Life of Alfred Schutz

Alfred Schutz's story – his history and his context – is relevant for understanding both the article he wrote and why the concepts in it become so deeply evident in the experiences of clinical ethicists. Schutz wrote "The Stranger: an Essay in Social Psychology" five years after he had emigrated to the US via Paris in order to escape the Nazi regime in Austria. Banker by trade, scholar by orientation, Schutz studied philosophy and sociology and began teaching part-time almost as soon as he arrived in New York in 1939 (while working on Wall Street). He taught at what had been the German University in Exile, which then became the New School for Social Research.

### Schutz's Stranger as a Model

It was in that context that Schutz wrote the essay, "The Stranger: An Essay in Social Psychology," which sets out to explore how an outsider, coming into a new group, attempts "to interpret the cultural pattern of [that] group … and to orient himself"[6] so as to be able to live within it and become part of it. Rather than investigating the challenges of leaving one's home group or the later process of assimilation, Schutz focuses on the Stranger's approach: difficult, disruptive, even dangerous at times, and thus requiring significant attention and effort. Schutz outlines the disruption experienced by the approaching Stranger, and the rigor and disciplined focus required as the Stranger seeks to understand this new "in-group" to which he does not yet belong but with whom he must engage: a process with striking parallels to clinical ethics work.

"The Stranger" is a broad example of several things, including what happens when your way of understanding the world around you shifts. The basis for that understanding was outlined by

Schutz in several other essays published around the same time as "The Stranger," which can help clarify the relevance of the Stranger's activities to clinical ethics practice. The key for Schutz was that the "world of working as a whole stands out as paramount."[7] This world of working is a world of action, and these elements are ones that we encounter in clinical work. Schutz explains:

> It is the world of physical things, including my body; it is the realm of my locomotions and bodily operations; it offers resistances that require effort to overcome; it places tasks before me, permits me to carry through my plans, and enables me to succeed or fail in my attempts to attain my purposes. By my working acts I gear into the outer world, I change it; and these changes, although provoked by my working, can be experienced and tested both by myself and others, as occurrences within this world independently of my working act in which they originated.[8]

It is because this "world of working is the reality within which communication and the interplay of mutual motivation becomes effective" that it is both shared by the Strangers and others, and communications and meanings can be tested. This is the world where the Stranger confronts the differences and modifications in the domains of new and different sets of actions and interpretations. They face a group of people going about their regular lives or engaging in particular projects or activities using widely understood and shared "recipes" – patterns of thought, action, and communication – that are accepted as routine and usual ways of thinking, acting, and speaking in order to get through the day or to complete particular projects.[9, 10, 11, 12] Schutz explains that recipes are handed down and absorbed from community life – from the graves of our grandfathers – such that they do not require (and more strongly, do not encourage or at times even allow) questioning about the whys and wherefores behind and underneath and woven into these recipes. Think Leonard Cohen's song "Everybody Knows" or Shirley Jackson's novella "We Have Always Lived in the Castle": in every community, there are some recipes, some understandings that members do not probe – or that members actively discourage probing. Depending on their history and potency, these recipes are just accepted and known as the way things work, the way things are, and the way things *should* be. The approaching Stranger, on the other hand, does *not* share this worldview and must piece together a functional understanding through observations and interactions. Such tentative and urgent work is required when one comes into a new environment, a new context, a new life-world. Even if that new world appears similar to one's own, it may still be significantly different: think here of an immigrant, arriving in an environment in which language, attire, social manners, food, *everything* is neither the same *nor* completely different from where they used to live. Whether immigrant or exile, the Stranger is not simply a visitor; they have been uprooted and come to live in this new culture, this new world, and so must learn what counts as "taken for granted," the typical "thinking as usual,"[13] and what serves as the "believed-in" reality. And, in the confrontation with all that is different in this new place, the exile also is confronted with what they "believed in" and took for granted up to now. They are not only a stranger as seen by those into whose world and culture they have landed, but they become a Stranger to their own prior world, to their own previous self *to what had been believed in.* The sense of "being a stranger" emerges in a more inward way, in a recognition, a sense of oneself as now different, even unfamiliar. And yet, the sense of "being a stranger" is a deeply internal process of disruptions and recognitions, experienced and undergone *at the same time* as the Stranger's focus must be directed outward – as they gear into the world, acting deliberately and carefully amid all those taken-for-granted nuances in relation to those others.

Schutz describes the Stranger's experience in approaching the in-group and is mostly concerned with the Stranger's effort to live and act within a social world that is new.[14] There are several similarities between the Stranger's activities and those in clinical ethics work. Both the Stranger and the ethicist begin by engaging with the partially organized, action-focused patterns of knowledge and taken-for-grantedness of the world as well as the requirements for "thinking-as-usual." Schutz's essay works through several key themes that highlight both the experiences of and the orientation of the Stranger. One key, of course, is that the Stranger and ethicist must come to terms with the ways that disruptions may irrupt in the world of everyday life and transform the significance of what was "taken-for-granted."

## Mapping the Unfamiliar World

The approaching Stranger doesn't know which way to go at first, even when observing the actions and movements that seem effortless to members of the community or in-group. In-group members can operate at ease in their environment because no one within the in-group has to know about everything in their worldview in depth. To illustrate, Schutz uses the image of a topographical map as a metaphor for the types of knowledge.[15] Some understandings require specific and deep familiarity (for Schutz's map, the slender, high peaks and narrow, deep chasms); others appear as localized but still distinguishable points of interest (hills and valleys), moving toward the broad ranges that create the backdrops of the in-group's world of working that are taken for granted (the wide plains and sedimented riverbeds). This is the in-group's world, where community members know on which side of the street they are to drive and how to behave or what topics can be raised in mixed company – and what hierarchies and histories make the company mixed in the first place. Schutz explains that all of this is recognized, known as natural and usual, and taken for granted such that members of the in-group can move through the day with much of their lives on autopilot[16]: unreflective and comfortable in the patterns and expectations that make the group familiar and safe.

For the Stranger, the approached in-group and their world are neither familiar nor safe. They are realms of uncertainty and confusion, where the recipes the approaching Stranger brings from *their* home community may have no analogues, or even if they exist, the Stranger may be unable to use them adequately, raising a "crisis" that their system of tested recipes "reveals that its applicability is restricted to a specific historical situation."[17] Their frames and means of understanding and acting within *their world* may not map onto the territories and terrains in which they now find themselves. And yet, having approached or engaged the in-group for whatever reason (necessity or desire, beyond simple curiosity), to continue to approach and to act within the in-group's world, the Stranger must be committed to investigating, learning, understanding, and practicing within that world. As Schutz writes, the Stranger becomes the person "who has to place in question nearly everything that seems to be unquestionable to members of the approached group."[18]

To become the Stranger in a strange land requires a difficult balance of attention and probing, combined with circumspection and caution. Interactions with members of the in-group and engagement with projects and activities of shared interest require the Stranger to pay close attention and give careful accounts (to themselves as much as or more than to others) of what they understand and how they are operating in this strange new world. This shift in perspective is both necessary and disconcerting, as Schutz describes,

> Jumping from the stalls to the stage, so to speak, the former onlooker becomes a member of the cast, enters as a partner into social relations with his co-actors, and participates henceforth in the action in progress.[19]

Such attention requires diligence and vigilance, deliberate observation, and careful reflection to make sense of what the in-group members "know" instinctively. In addition, this shift from perception to action illustrates that these meanings are intersubjective, and as we will continue to explore throughout the chapters that follow in this book, this social world is "storied." Stories are the medium through which these meanings are managed and actions interpreted, so the Stranger must move around and be careful about the fringes of meaning and expectation that lurk below the surface of common speech and typical behaviors,[20] humbly seeking to understand the language, stories, and meanings of the new situation without stumbling into shibboleths of such magnitude that they risk ejection (whether of the polite or forceful variety) from the group. The Stranger's engagement with the taken-for-granted world of the approached in-group is one of never being quite at ease, always alert, attentive, vigilant – on edge, even – because the taken-for-granted working world for the in-group is a "field of actual and possible acts."[21] At the same time, for the Stranger, this field is full of unknown paths and not-always-clear options, and those motivations, acts, and stories become a challenge to interpret and understand.

On the other hand, Schutz points out that from their unknowing and the distance that allows for testing the "believed-in" meanings, not being already committed to the paths and options circumscribed by what is taken-for-granted enables the Stranger to also inhabit, literally enact, a perspective for critical engagement with the known and accepted cultural patterns of the in-group. They can see more clearly, at times, some of the structures and underlying values and commitments that may be invisible to members of the in-group – hidden and obscured by the weight of experience and history and "this is how things always work."[22] The clear eyes of the Stranger may help them navigate creatively and responsively through the strange land and deliberately and conscientiously engage with and respond to the thoughts, actions, and communications of the in-group members.

Schutz observes two deep roots for such a critical engagement. First is the "objective" aspect of the lived reality of the social world. Confronted in this way, the Stranger's "objectivity" stems from their deep need to pay attention to and understand what is going on in order to successfully manage their actions in the world of working. From expected greetings to acquiring food to learning how to avoid offending with inappropriate dress, the Stranger's observations must be both wide-ranging and keenly focused on similarities and differences from their previous experiences in order to adopt and make use of the accepted recipes in the taken-for-granted world of the in-group. Critical engagement is a practical need.

The second is a more reflective and thus, more personally challenging root of critical engagement. In the encounter, the Stranger faces uncomfortable and disruptive recognition of the partiality, idiosyncrasy, and limitations of their own experiences and their own recipes. Their trusted, historically and culturally validated ways of being in the world and taking the world for granted are suddenly less familiar and not as safe. Schutz explains,

> In other words, the cultural pattern of the approached group is to the Stranger not a shelter but a field of adventure, not a matter of course, but a questionable topic of investigation, not an instrument for disentangling problematic situations but a problematic situation itself and one hard to master.[23]

Their experience of being the Stranger is the awesome and discomfiting recognition that their home-country worldview may have *never* been safe or comfortable and likely will never be again. Thus, the Stranger's crucial engagement grows from realizing that their pride in navigating and mastering the world up until *now* may be valid *only* up to this point and that their recipes, skill, and knowledge may not be sufficient outside of their community of origin.[24]

The other source of the Stranger's unease is that their critical engagement is often met with surprise and suspicion by the approached group.[25] By not accepting the patterns of thought, action, and communication of the in-group unequivocally, the Stranger acquires the stigma of being, in

Schutz's phrase, the "marginal man" of doubtful loyalty. Members of the in-group are appalled and baffled by the Stranger's questioning of what their way *is*. The Stranger's questioning and the objectivity with which they consider the local gods and shibboleths of the approached group challenge the assurance that the in-group's way is the best way, the only way, and "the best of all possible solutions to any problem."[26] As Schutz explains,

> The Stranger is called ungrateful since he refuses to acknowledge that the cultural pattern offered to him grants him shelter and protection. But these people do not understand that the Stranger in a state of transition does not consider this pattern as a protecting shelter at all, but as a labyrinth in which he has lost all sense of his bearing.[27]

The Stranger, if they are paying attention at all (as they must always be) is constantly aware of their inter-relational and existential vulnerability: that they tread on thin ice, that their invitation or the welcome they received if the approach was theirs, can be and may be rescinded at a moment's notice, with or without explanation.

Thus, the Stranger's orientation and approach exhibit elements of responsibility that are key to their interactions: coming to terms with disruption and the need for careful attention; the demand for self-reflection; affiliation with others and its concomitant ongoing vulnerability; and recognition of the ways telling stories opens into that sometimes difficult creation of meaning from different understandings, especially when they appear to matter so deeply. The Stranger approaches with *care* because they seek to understand and interact with the in-group – to walk with them, live with them, and engage with their projects – for however long and for whatever purpose. The Stranger must *take care* and be responsible for themselves: aware of and responsive to their own vulnerability. Equally important, the Stranger must *take care* of those they approach. The Stranger does not come as an iconoclast or recklessly and authoritatively to show these others the error of their ways. The Stranger seeks to engage the approached group for whatever mutual purpose, whatever shared circumstance is at hand – which means respecting and acknowledging the power and resonance of the in-group's taken-for-granted stories about being in the world. At the same time, the Stranger's very presence may disrupt them, unintentionally, or the Stranger may discover in the encounter that the circumstances of the mutual projects and activities may require that the in-group must be deliberately disrupted or challenged by thinking differently and incorporating each other's pre-existing recipes. The Stranger must do so *carefully* and *deliberately,* however, with concern not just for their safety and continued engagement but with and from the remembrance and experience of one who has been similarly challenged and disrupted.

Schutz ends his powerful and eloquent essay by noting that the *process* of the Stranger acclimating into a new social group occurs in other spheres of human engagement, too, and "are general categories of our interpretation of the world."[28] As humans, we move between categories of strangeness and familiarity in the everyday as well as in our encounters with the uncanny. We approach the unfamiliar with "a process of inquiry," trying to bring the strange into coherence with our previous knowledge, experiences, and activities. The process described by Schutz is so ubiquitous that we rarely think about it for long because "if we succeed in this endeavor, then that which formerly was a strange fact and a puzzling problem to our mind is transformed into an additional element of our wanted knowledge."[29] The new information we acquire in our strangeness helps build new recipes, new approaches, and new responses that fit within the expanded world as we *now* know it and in the cultural patterns of the new community.

Schutz closes by observing that if this process of inquiry is successful, the unfamiliar "pattern and its elements will become to the newcomer a matter of course, an unquestionable way of life, a shelter and a protection," at which point, per Schutz, "the 'Stranger' is no stranger anymore and his specific problem has been solved."[30] We then face something else entirely, a different set of "problems," perhaps other questions. But as they assimilate, the Stranger can loosen their tight attention and relax out of their disease into a better understood, more readily familiar world of working within the in-group.

## The Stranger's Discipline and Elements of Responsibility in Clinical Ethics

So, the question emerges right here, at the beginning of this book: why would I, why do I suggest there is value in recognizing this role as a Stranger? More pointedly, how, or why, would recognition of this sort of disruption experienced by being a Stranger be a crucial element of clinical ethics practice? After all, Schutz seems to paint a fairly challenging picture of the Stranger's experiences – a tale of, if not outright woe, at least one of real everyday trials and even tribulations. The Stranger's challenges are multi-faceted: unknowing and uncertainty, anxiety and risk, concern for others and concern for self, the urgent need to understanding with sharp awareness that understanding may not come in time – or at all. For Schutz, the Stranger approaching the in-group seeks assimilation and understanding: trading the strangeness for familiarity seems to be the goal. So why introduce and then advocate for a clinical ethics practice that suggests the discipline of strangeness is important to keep in mind when what is offered appears to be such disruptive experiences of uncertainty and risk? What is the value of an orientation that demands perpetual distancing and constant vigilance?

It's a fair question – and one with which I and my mentors are familiar. As Richard M. Zaner, a student of Schutz and my teacher's teacher, exclaims about clinical ethics practice, "Who in their right mind would invite someone into this?"[31] Or, as my teacher, Mark J. Bliton pointed out during my clinical ethics training, "If you can do anything else you probably should ..." Which he followed by observing, "... but by the time you realize it, it is probably too late." Once you encounter these kinds of questions and human experiences, you may not be able to look away. You may be caught by the wonder: what is this like and how do people live through this (whatever *this* is)? As Bliton notes, "... ingredient in the activities and familiarity of moral experience in ethics consultations is the individual's discovery of his/her humanity – and the fact that he or she may lack real and important knowledge about what that means."[32] And with that disruption and recognition comes the Stranger's question: how do *I* do this? How do I find out, navigate, learn, and live in this strange land?

Working from within, out of, and through my tradition, the compulsion to understand and make sense of the uncanny in settings of illness and injury, caring for and being cared for by others sees the work of clinical ethics as deliberately taking on the activities of the Stranger. Clinical ethics consultation is a process of embarking on projects of understanding and sense-making with other strangers in their in-groups and as they approach other in-groups themselves, by invitation, accident, or necessity. Clinical ethics requires being open to being disrupted by other people's concerns, commitments, histories, thoughts, actions, and modes of communication that comprise *their* recipes for being in the world. Navigating their disruption as the Stranger *in the role as a clinical ethics consultant* also provides a model for others in the clinical encounter.

When the clinical ethics consultant is invited into a clinical situation, it is because some of the people involved, some among the groups already present, have become strangers – often unwillingly and often unavoidably, through the illness or injury of themselves or a loved one. They have become strangers to themselves, to their community, their ways of being in the world; their frames and recipes for interpreting meanings and making sense of the world are inadequate. They are *different* ... in ways that they may not yet understand. The patients, families, and clinicians who call the clinical ethics consultant for help or support are in the crisis of the Stranger – suddenly uncertain: attentive, vulnerable, forced to engage with other strangers, and perhaps to reconsider all they hold true and dear and real. Disruption can be a tool for clinical ethics consultants, as for the Stranger, enabling them to expand their encounters with and understanding of recipes for being in the world.

People in clinical settings experience this crisis in circumstances that demand action, often with limited time, and that may carry ultimate consequences: a radically altered or even ended life. The shearing disruption and "fundamental anxiety" of these strange experiences make being a Stranger unavoidable for some, perhaps all, of those involved. The primary stakeholders (in ethics-speak) are the people with whom the ethics consultant engages: those with some skin in the game, for whom these circumstances and consequences matter, and for whom the options and choices are real, "live options," in William James's phrase.[33] Healthcare settings are strange lands indeed, where many – even most – may be struggling and stumbling through the problems and experiences of a Stranger in forced circumstances, at warp speed, and with little preparation. They are the ones who find themselves estranged from their everyday modes of being and acting. So why, amid all this disruption, discerning, and potential despair, should the clinical ethics consultant deliberately take on the activities and orientation of the Stranger?

The impetus and moral compulsion for ethics consultants to *take on the orientation of the Stranger* is because they *can* – and can do so in service to the consultation and those who have become strangers without choosing. The clinical ethics consultant knows what it is to be a stranger in a strange land – and has discovered that strangeness *can* offer clarity and possibility even in the disruption of unknowing and the sudden instability of previously held recipes for action. Although any given moment of a clinical encounter is new and unique to the ethics consultant as Stranger, the elements of disruption run throughout. As the Stranger's experience of disruption becomes familiar, they can walk through disruption with others who may be less practiced and with more at stake in the circumstances, choices, and potential aftermaths. The ethics consultant's disciplined orientation as Stranger is their unique ability to care for others in whom they recognize a similar estrangement from what they knew and how they used to do.

The ethics consultant accepts responsibility through the role[34] as resource/service/help/support, depending on local or institutional expectations, but their responsibility presents and emerges in their activities, especially their ability to intentionally practice and even model the strategic, savvy, critical engagement Schutz describes. From their slight remove or near distance to the crisis requiring their involvement, the ethics consultant can engage in a close reading of the situation and paying attention to "what's going on": here, now, for and with the people in the bed, at bedside, in the community. The ethics consultant meets the challenge of accounting for their questions and probing, as coming from a need to understand; they experience deep vulnerability as their own commitments (recipes, beliefs, and sense of self) come into question and require strenuous self-reflection. And all this occurs through the intentional willingness to face the unknowing and uncertainty with people wrapped up and swept under by it. The ethics consultant's critical engagement *as the Stranger* may allow them the objectivity (in Schutz's term) to see options and possibilities, to ask questions, and to probe understandings otherwise unfathomable to those caught and surrendered to their own crisis. True, such probing and questioning may put the ethics consultant at risk of being dis-invited from future engagements or ejected from one of the groups with whom they are engaged. Their risk and potential consequences, however, are significantly less than those threatening the other stakeholders, those primarily involved in the clinical situation at hand, at least at the outset of the circumstance sparking the consultant's engagement.

When the ethics consultant takes on the activities and orientation of the Stranger in a deliberate and explicit way, they must first recognize and respond to their disruption and the *strangeness* of the circumstances in which they find themselves. In recognizing that strangeness, they *may be able to engage,* intentionally and proactively, in the behaviors Schutz describes. In the Stranger's discipline and orientation, they have a real, live chance of responding *responsibly* to whatever circumstances are at hand, though such engagement is not, however, guaranteed. Nor is learning or understanding or welcome from the in-group, for that matter, no matter how disciplined the approach of the ethics consultant as Stranger. Even without the guarantee, however, Schutz's vivid and detailed description of the Stranger's experience and discipline provides a frame and a language for articulating an important element of clinical ethics consultation practice.

### *What's So Strange About a Seminar?*

Years later, I can see the parallel lessons of Schutz's description of the Stranger and of Seminar. They both informed and still shape my clinical practice – especially around understanding the inherent disruption of what I do. Yet the differences are important too. The Stranger aims for eventual assimilation into the in-group which, as Schutz notes, carries its own collection of challenges.[35] The Stranger, even in their disruption, seeks a restoration of balance, incorporating local flavors and traditions into their beloved recipes and taken-for-granted ways of being in the world. The Stranger aiming toward assimilation learns to drive on the correct side of the road and how not to offend the local gods – by accident or intent. I also learned, however, that the work doesn't necessarily end in a Stranger's assimilation to the new ways of being and acting.

The Stranger offers the same striking lesson as Seminar: the rigor of disruption and the orientation to strangeness are never ending. In clinical ethics and clinical philosophy, the disruption is ongoing and requires just as much attention, rigor, and tolerance for uncertainty twenty years into my career as it did twenty minutes into the first class on the first day. Seminar became a method for learning about deep elements of responsibility in clinical ethics practice – by undergoing the moral experience of the Stranger with other strangers. Each element – disruption, attention, self-reflection, attunement, recognition of vulnerability, and a willingness to share our own stories – was part of an intentionally reflexive discipline encountered, articulated, and demonstrated in Seminar. These elements of responsibility – and the practice of intentionally engaging in them with others – have structured and supported my work in clinical ethics and clinical philosophy long after the Seminar ended.

The practices of Seminar remain relevant as a deeply engaging method of clinical ethics work and as a means of engagement with the clinical context: concerned with the deep, elemental, and interpersonal questions of being human in bodies that exceed our choices and control from before birth to death and beyond, requiring care for, care by, and care with other humans. The efforts of Schutz's Stranger, along with the practice clinical philosophy developed from Seminar (or whichever iteration/version of Seminar existed at other institutions), persist as orientations and activities that can be identified, described, articulated, modeled, and practiced.

These elements of practice offer neither a script nor a stepwise algorithm – they are not tied to one program or particular framework for clinical ethics. Rather, these efforts toward understanding and elements of responsible practice emerge in local contexts and institutional dynamics: a thread linking experiences across different encounters. Like improvisational dance, they allow fluid movement practiced in real time; or like the oral traditions of storytelling, or call and answer of folksongs, all those involved make the chorus richer, bringing out the details in their questions and replies. Through the ethics consultant's deliberate practice and the discipline of Schutz's Stranger, those dances, those stories and songs, *are* ongoing, *are still* being created in interpersonal interactions among and between communities and strangers, and as such, they remain sources for and opportunities for mutual learning, reflection, and practice.

# Notes

1 Churchill, Larry R. (1978). "The ethicist in professional education." *Hastings Center Report* 8 (6):13–15.
2 Barnard, David (1992). "Reflections of a reluctant clinical ethicist: Ethics consultation and the collapse of critical distance." *Theoretical Medicine and Bioethics* 13 (1):15–22.
3 Tiryakian, Edward A. (1973) "Sociological perspectives on the stranger." *Soundings: An Interdisciplinary Journal* 5 (1):45–58.
4 Agich, George J. (1990). "Clinical ethics: A role theoretic look." *Social Science & Medicine* 30 (4):389–399.
5 Schutz, Alfred (1944). "The stranger: An essay in social psychology." *American Journal of Sociology* 49 (6):499–507.
6 *Ibid.* 499.
7 Schutz, Alfred (1962). "On Multiple Realities." In Maurice Natanson (ed.), *Collected Papers of Alfred Schutz: The Problem of Social Reality*, vol 1. The Hague: Martinus Nijhoff. p. 226.
8 *Ibid.* 226–227.
9 Schutz, *The Stranger*, 501.
10 Natanson, Maurice (1962). "Introduction." In Maurice Natanson (ed.), *Collected Papers of Alfred Schutz: The Problem of Social Reality*, vol 1, XXV–XLVII. The Hague: Martinus Nijhoff. pp. 24–26.
11 Schutz, Alfred (1962). "Some Leading Concepts in Phenomenology" In Maurice Natanson (ed.), *Collected Papers of Alfred Schutz: The Problem of Social Reality*, vol 1. The Hague: Martinus Nijhoff. pp. 99–117.
12 James, William (1975). *Pragmatism.* Cambridge, MA: Harvard University Press. pp. 74–75.
13 Schutz, *The Stranger*, 501.
14 *Ibid.* 499.
15 *Ibid.* 500.
16 *Ibid.* 501.
17 *Ibid.* 502.
18 *Ibid.* 502.
19 *Ibid.* 503.
20 *Ibid.* 504–505.
21 *Ibid.* 500.
22 *Ibid.* 504.
23 *Ibid.* 506.
24 This is part of what forms a deep challenge to the professionalization and standardization in the field of clinical ethics and that against which it struggles most vehemently: the Stranger's stark and sobering recognition that their own truth is no less provincial and partial than anyone else's. The appalling humility such an outrageous recognition demands presents as an utter betrayal of expertise – a refutation of the idea of *mastery* – of concrete, generalizable knowledge. The Stranger's deliberate and "bitter acceptance" of their limitations is an affront to totalizing forces of authority and hierarchy – political and epistemological and moral (even those at play in the field of clinical ethics). The Stranger knows they cannot make ultimate or final assertions in the domain of honest and open engagement with others.
25 Schutz, *The Stranger*, 506–507.
26 *Ibid.* 507.
27 *Ibid.*
28 *Ibid.* 507.
29 *Ibid.*
30 *Ibid.*
31 Bartlett, Virginia L., Bartlett, Shane K., Bliton, Mark J., and Finder, Stuart G. (2015). *The Oral History of Healthcare Ethics: Volume 1 – A Life in Clinical Philosophy: A Conversation with Richard M. Zaner.* Video available: http://ohhe.org
32 Bliton, Mark J. (2008). "Maternal-Fetal Surgery and the 'Profoundest Question in Ethics'" In P.J. Ford and D.M. Dudzinski (eds.), *Complex Ethics Consultations: Cases That Haunt Us*. Cambridge: Cambridge University Press. p. 40.
33 James, William (1918). *The Principles of Psychology.* New York: H. Holt and Company. pp. 296–297.
34 Finder, Stuart G., and Bliton, Mark J. (2001). "Activities, not rules: The need for responsive practice (on the way toward responsibility)." *American Journal of Bioethics* 1 (4):52–54.
35 Schutz, *The Stranger*, 507.

## Bibliography

Agich, George J. (1990). "Clinical ethics: A role theoretic look." *Social Science & Medicine* 30 (4):389–399.

Barnard, David (1992). "Reflections of a reluctant clinical ethicist: Ethics consultation and the collapse of critical distance." *Theoretical Medicine and Bioethics* 13 (1):15 22.

Bartlett, Virginia L., Bartlett, Shane K., Bliton, Mark J., and Finder, Stuart G. (2015). *The Oral History of Healthcare Ethics: Volume 1 – A Life in Clinical Philosophy: A Conversation with Richard M. Zaner*. Video available: http://ohhe.org

Bliton, Mark J. (2008). "Maternal-Fetal Surgery and the 'Profoundest Question in Ethics'" In P.J. Ford and D.M. Dudzinski (eds.), *Complex Ethics Consultations: Cases That Haunt Us*. Cambridge: Cambridge University Press..

Churchill, Larry R. (1978). "The ethicist in professional education." *Hastings Center Report* 8 (6):13–15.

Finder, Stuart G., and Bliton, Mark J. (2001). "Activities, not rules: The need for responsive practice (on the way toward responsibility)." *American Journal of Bioethics* 1 (4):52–54..

James, William (1918). *The Principles of Psychology*. New York: H. Holt and Company. pp. 296–297.

James, William (1975). *Pragmatism*. Cambridge, MA: Harvard University Press. pp. 74–75.

Natanson, Maurice (1962). "Introduction." In Maurice Natanson (ed.), *Collected Papers of Alfred Schutz: The Problem of Social Reality*, vol 1, XXV–XVLII. The Hague: Martinus Nijhoff. pp. 24–26.

Schutz, Alfred (1944). The Stranger: An Essay in Social Psychology. *American Journal of Sociology* 49 (6):499–507.

Schutz, Alfred. (1962). "On Multiple Realities." In Maurice Natanson (ed.), *Collected Papers of Alfred Schutz: The Problem of Social Reality*, vol 1. The Hague: Martinus Nijhoff.

Schutz, Alfred (1962). "Some Leading Concepts in Phenomenology." In Maurice Natanson (ed.), *Collected Papers of Alfred Schutz: The Problem of Social Reality*, vol 1. The Hague: Martinus Nijhoff. pp. 99–117.

Tiryakian, Edward A. (1973). "Sociological perspectives on the stranger." *Soundings: An Interdisciplinary Journal* 5 (1):45–58.

# 2    Clinical Attention as Surrender-and-Catch

**Mr. Jones and Me**

There was shit smeared everywhere.

When the patient's legs jackknifed across the bed, the sheet flew up and I felt revulsion ripple across my face. I glanced around, afraid someone would notice. No one was looking at me. I saw David's face mirror what mine must have looked like and felt a moment's camaraderie, however one sided. He clamped his lips tight, controlled, and reached down to pull the sheet back over, flat, tucking it under knees and feet on the bed to cover the mess.

I followed David's lead, schooling my face into what I hoped was a neutral and impassive curiosity. My teeth ground together until my jaw ached, but I suspected that if my reactions were too noticeable, someone would look at me. And might ask me to leave the patient's room. And I didn't want to leave. Despite the stench. Despite the deep soul-blush of seeing a stranger's scrotum and butt, blotchy with infection and covered with shit.

Back and forth, I kept looking at the others, the faces of the others in the room: David and the other residents, Dr. Wiley with his wavy hair and focused gaze. The nurse, peeling back the corners of sterile pads and packets of swabs that she placed on a tray near the bed.

Back and forth. I cringed inward with the shame of an unintentional voyeur, an illegitimate trespasser, afraid of being found out, afraid of expulsion. How did I get here? I pull back my shoulders and put my breath into staying: this is how I'll learn.

\*\*\*

"hmmmmm … dammmit."

The murmur is so faint I craned my head to see if it was the patient or Dr. Wiley, who is known for both his attention-pulling *sotto voce* and his crescendoed bellow to the residents who do not meet their responsibilities.

"HOME I WANT GO GODDAMMIT"

My eyes whipped back down to the bed where the patient danced himself across the blue and white chux pads. Too weak to pull himself upright, he scrunched over neck to knees, his chin jutting over his shin. I saw his shape frozen in time, a grotesque in a Bosch triptych.

Hands and voices rushed to soothe him, straightening the sheets he kept kicking off, smoothing his stringy hair. A nasal, mountain twang jolted my attention again.

"Luke, we'll get you home but you gotta let these doctors look at you."

The woman brushing his hair back from his sweaty forehead carried the same sharp features he did, framed by blonde waves and bangs of the "higher the hair, the closer to Jesus" sort.

DOI: 10.4324/9781003354864-4

This woman's drawl continued, in pace with her hand on the patient's forehead: "He didn't want to come in, but I made him. I knew he was in a bad way."

Dr. Wiley, asked, "Is he your brother?" She nodded. "Can you tell me what happened?"

The blonde woman snuffled back tears and looked at the man standing beside her. "You tell him, Bill," she said, and nodded to Dr. Wiley. "Bill's my husband."

Bill dragged his eyes away from the bed, where his brother-in-law squinched his eyes down into his sunken cheeks.

"He got fired on Friday, Doc," Bill began. "He came home with a pink slip and a case of beer, and we started drinking before dinner. I went on home when it got dark, but Luke was still on the porch with half a case to go."

Dr. Wiley listened hard, and with palpable kindness as he sat on the edge of the bed, his hand resting on the patient's feet. Bill continued.

"I walked over Saturday morning to check on him, but he wasn't in the house. I walked around the side, by the porch, and found him out by the wood pile – passed out cold. Best he could remember was stepping off the porch to take a piss. I guess he fell down and stayed down. Good thing it ain't too cold yet. Anyway, I took him in and got him into bed. He came over Sunday and didn't look right and he kept scratching – said he had a bite on his hip. Leslie here didn't think he looked good at all and made him show her what he was pickin' at."

Leslie broke into the story. "He wouldn't listen to me. It looked awful – dark in the middle and red spreading all around. He said he was just hungover and all he needed was some aspirin and some calamine lotion. He went back home, but I checked on him last night and he was on the couch, shaking and sweating with fever and I told him we were coming up to the hospital this morning and I didn't give a damn what he said. I told them all this down in emergency and they sent him right up here."

She held everyone in the rhythm of the story and when she paused, it was as if a freeze-framed video released, noise and bustle resuming. Luke moaned again: "nahmo fussin" came out as one jumbled word, catching on a thickened tongue.

Dr. Wiley patted Luke's foot and thanked Leslie and Bill for filling him in and getting Luke to the hospital. "So, he maybe got bitten on Friday night? And fever getting worse for … let's see, it's Monday, so almost three days?"

They nodded, and Bill put his hand on Leslie's shoulder and squeezed. Dr. Wiley nodded in return and asked them to step out and into the hallway so he and the residents could look at Luke. Leslie smoothed Luke's hair one more time before she and Bill walked to the door.

I was watching Luke, Mr. Jones, still writhing and mouthing "mmmfine. Just … home" when I heard the heavy grey door thud shut. The room was suddenly emptier than it had been.

\*\*\*

I glanced around again and realized the pharmacy residents and the librarian from the medical library were gone. They had followed the family into the hallway. Dr. Wiley was looking at me and I felt my eyes hold the unasked question. Everyone in that room had a reason to be there, except for me. Something to do for Mr. Jones, for Luke. Should I go? Or should I stay? Dr. Wiley held my gaze and gave me nothing. Not a nod, a raised eyebrow, not a shrug. I had to decide. And I stayed. He turned away, and I watched the sudden burst of activity.

The nurse gave the residents supplies and went to get test tubes, to lay beside the swabs on the tray. Dr. Wiley stretched on blue gloves he'd pulled from a box on the wall over by the sink. David and Tim, another resident, rolled Mr. Jones on his right side, so he faced them, giving Dr. Wiley, another resident named Sheri, the fellow, and the nurse a clear view. I stood off to the side, a little behind the wall of white-clad shoulders that were now standing by or bent over or crouched to the floor at the side of the bed. When my gaze traveled from the shifting lab coats to Luke, my focus was resolute.

Mess. What a mess. The phrase pulsed in my mind. His flesh was a mess. The bacteria had made a mess of his flesh. He had lesions and pus-filled boils on his buttocks and deeply flushed – almost purple – splotches crawling over his skin toward his hip bone. As dark as the splotches were, there seemed to be an odd transparency about them – almost as if I could see how deep the infection went into is body – stained glass skin. There were lava-red splits along the wrinkled skin of his scrotum. Rot. Mess. Ooze. Shit. I don't think I breathed until I saw David grimace, peering over Mr. Jones's side, as he held a steady grip on shoulder and ribcage.

He'd gone quiet now, like he was unaware of the fellow and Dr. Wiley, who were pressing and prodding his skin, pulling it from side to side. Mr. Jones grasped dazedly at the papers in David's lab coat, right at eye level, just through the bedrails. David lifted the papers out of Mr. Jones's fingers and gently put the wandering hand back on the mattress where it gripped and tangled the sheets.

My fascination broke as I felt eyes on me again. I looked back at the doctors, expecting to see Dr. Wiley's evaluative scrutiny. Instead, it was Sheri, now sitting in the chair by the wall. She was watching me, but gave no acknowledgement, no curiosity, no smile. Nothing but a blank gaze that shifted to David, to the fellow, to the nurse. Everywhere except the patient. Her face froze for a moment when her gaze met Dr. Wiley's and it was as if he led her gaze back to Mr. Jones and his weeping sores.

That weight of Dr. Wiley's attention settled on me for a moment. I again felt the push-pull of cringing inward, into myself and mute outreach: what am I doing here? Please let me stay. I spoke neither out loud. Dr. Wiley shifted his surveillance, all the while explaining to the residents what he was doing in each physical action. He pulled loose a swab from the sterile plastic wrapper, which fell to the floor, its protection no longer necessary.

"For something like this level of infection, you want the long handle, because you're going to be feeling for the depth of necrosis." All eyes followed Dr. Wiley's voice to the suddenly powerful looking instrument.

While Dr. Wiley pointed to the largest lesion, the fellow held apart its edges so the probe went in carefully. Mr. Jones didn't seem to notice, and a tinge of horror shivered through my focus as I realized how much of the wooden handle had disappeared below the skin.

"The tissue is dead most of the way down to the bone, which is why Luke here isn't reacting much. It makes it easier to do this, but isn't a good sign. This means the infection is deep and wide. We need to culture this and get his antibiotics narrowed as quickly as we can, and call for plastic surgery to schedule a debridement." Mr. Jones screamed.

"Stop … leamelone … ahhooooowwww." His voice was thick and slurry, like a drunk's. He tried again: "Want go-home, dammit."

Dr. Wiley gave one last swirl of the swab and pulled it out. My eyes flicked between the patient and the sample. David took over for Leslie and smoothed back Luke's hair with one hand while he held Luke's torso firm and steady with the other. Dr. Wiley plunged the gooey end of the swab into the test tube, held at the ready by the nurse. She clipped the excess handle with a snapping sound and popped on the rubber top to seal it. It was a ballet of efficiency, clinical choreography engrained in muscle memory. Sheri and I looked at each other and our eyes bounced away: the moment too raw to share with a stranger.

Mr. Jones's voice had lowered to a drawling mutter, somewhere between a mosquito whine and a growl. David and Tim helped roll him from his side to his back and straightened the sheets around him. Dr. Wiley had removed his gloves and was using the foot pedals to operate the scrub sink – splitting his attention between cleaning his hands up past his wrists and asking the nurse to page him when the lab results came back. She nodded, "Of course, Dr. Wiley," as she cleaned and straightened up all around the bed, picking up the wrapper from the sterile swab.

Mr. Jones, Luke, burrowed his shoulders into the flat pillow and held onto the sheets by his side, balling them into his fist. Brown seeped through by his fingers. I wanted to point out the mess to someone, but, still unsure of my role, unsure of whether I should have even been there at all, if I had any right to make suggestions or ask such questions, I didn't speak up. I followed as everyone left the room except Mr. Jones.

## Never Quite Easy Again: The Surrender of Attention, the Surrender-To of Paying Attention

### *Disruption and Attention in Clinical Contexts*

After the Mr. Jones encounter, I began to explore of the experience of disruption and the ways aspects of disruption were continually present in clinical ethics work. By disruption, I mean abrupt, unchosen shifts of attention: finding oneself jolted from an intentional focus on things understood or pursued from within previous frames of understanding to a seemingly inescapable shift of attention to something, some person, some moment that exceeds prior experience. While there are many elements of clinical ethics available for consideration in the story of Mr. Jones, what stands out most clearly are the deep shifts of attention and intentions which grow from the experience of disruption. The focused attention and deliberate observations I had intended to bring to my clinical rounds in the Medical Intensive Care Unit (MICU) shifted, like they went somewhere else, startled and stunned by my encounters in the drama of that situation. I was thrown by a sense of strangeness, uncertainty, and an urgency to understand, not merely because the circumstance was disconcerting in its newness and visceral elements, but because, like Alfred Schutz's Stranger,[1] my taken-for-granted, typical recipes for understanding a situation felt not just out of place, but alarmingly inadequate.

This is one of the first really sharp-in-memory "moment of disruption" where my attention was captured rather than directed, and crucial to note because such experiences have been present in nearly every clinical ethics consult I have responded to since. Recognizing the shifting boundaries in attentional control – and the experience of being deliberately attentive, even to these shifts – showed the ways that what I had taken-for-granted moved into the background as newer, insistent aspects enforced a focus on what was not readily incorporated into my previous experience. Exemplified starkly with Mr. Jones, the vivid fixing of attention combined with heightened awareness that I had little idea about what was actually happening shifted my focus of attention to *how I was paying attention* in that moment.

Recognizing the importance of paying attention to my own attention – especially while in such moments that disrupt prior expectations and assumptions - also raised the question of how I *had been* paying attention in previous, mundane moments. It meant acknowledging, somehow, that these facets of disruption seem recurrent, if not ubiquitous: I faced an unwelcome reality that I was not as in control of my attention as I had presumed, less even than I would have imagined. And yet, I still held some idea that with enough education and acquired knowledge, with enough careful attention and focus, I could know and understand the "*real* ethics issues" in an encounter.

Before my encounter with Mr. Jones (and long after, it turns out), I carried a deep concern that if I wasn't intentional about what I was learning, if I was disrupted and "thrown back on myself," I would be "doing it wrong." I worried that these experiences of disruption, of being thrown off-kilter and having my attention drawn and pulled meant I wasn't being "clinical" enough. How could I possibly be disrupted after such careful practice and preparation and self-reflection – in Seminar? With my teachers? Throughout the earlier days of rounds? What if I was so disrupted I wouldn't be able to understand or make sense of all that was going on? In looking back at the documents of my early training – journals, reflections, and papers – my questions about these elements of being disrupted were rooted in some strong commitments, expecting my clinical ethics training to be something linear, something progressive. I presumed that as I learned more I could more deliberately, even effectively, participate, that I could focus on "real" ethics issues, not just pinballing from one disconcerting experience to another. I wanted there to be a sense of mastery, competence – a real shift from "when I was a child a spoke like a child" to "now I have put away childish things." And how could it be otherwise? Those expectations (and desires) were part of the educational scaffolding that had gotten me from high school to college to graduate school. I can see (now) why I was so committed to finding a stepwise frame to manage whatever came next in my clinical exposures: rounds, Seminar, reflective writings.

### Mr. Jones and the Experience of Surrender

Even in those early moments of my training, however, a frame of incremental mastery did not accommodate or account for the staggering disruptions that followed, even prior to standing dumbfounded by Mr. Jones's bedside. Throughout my training journal, I find experiences of being thrown by encountering something deeply *other* and unknown, with the constant strangeness of "What is this?" "What now?" "What's next?," and "What is going on?" emerging on every page. However, each experience seemed to be manageable with deliberate attention and investigation, moving into or approaching with tools, "recipes" (in Schutz's term) for making sense of the world. Now, after months of trying to focus, and practicing, intentionally interrogating everything I saw in the MICU, not being in control of my attention in the moments with Mr. Jones was unnerving. It seemed personal.

Like the disruptive recognition in Seminar that knowledge acquisition and skill mastery weren't adequate, in the halls of the MICU, no matter where I looked, I couldn't find the Bioethics theories I'd read about: autonomy, beneficence, do no harm. None of it was even in the language, the vocabularies or communications of others in the MICU. I felt like Minnie Driver's character in the movie, *Grosse Pointe Blank*: "Shut up about the theories! I don't care about the theories! I want to know about the dead people. EXPLAIN the dead people."[2] Mr. Jones wasn't dead, but his injury and illness were inescapably compelling – to me and the others in the room; his physical needs, his and his family's uncertainty and distress, the experiences of the clinicians – the other trainees – they carried a similar need to be understood. And that could not be intellectualized away, at least not in the moment. For me, the raw experience was not cognitive or empirical – it was concrete and interpersonal, shared and interactive. Mr. Jones's body twitched and my gut clenched in response. David's face shape-shifted through a welter of emotions and expressions – and I could feel mine dancing in its own waves of activations. Sheri's eyes darted to and drilled down into others' faces and movements – as did mine – and when our laser beam gazes crossed paths, the pause was electric in its sympathy and pulsed with challenges before they separated again. In the overwhelm of the encounter, *this* moment, I *questioned everything*, even as I tried to take in, gather more to learn in everything. I was overcome by the uncertainties even in the ways I question, how I take things in at *any* moment. Analysis and application of theories seemed remote, as if the vivid humanity and drama created a kind of distance, and that kind of clinical comeuppance to my valued intellectual preparation was disconcerting.

### Intellectualizing the Disruption Away

You see, I had been working steadily and conscientiously to make sense of and master the context and concerns of the MICU (though I didn't recognize that's what I was attempting to do at the time, nor did I have any idea *why* I thought that was expected). I came into rounds with an intentional and studied openness – begun in the work of Seminar – as a practiced curiosity, and with a deep interest of several years standing. I carried my awareness of my trepidation like an amulet, protective, as if by admitting the things I was nervous about or afraid of, I would only encounter those. I used what I knew like a fire break – dug in as borders to keep the edges of the maelstrom just far enough away. But sometimes ash and sparks fly farther than one expects – and Mr. Jones was a burning tree that crashed near me and sent unanticipated recognitions and difficult questions firing off toward new horizons.

The fire metaphor reads as extreme, perhaps, but on the other hand, the disruption was profound in ways that exceeded the encounter. The existential experience of those brief moments reverberate down through my clinical training and experience as so pivotal. All the curiosity and preparation and intention in the world may – or may not – be enough to make sense of, understand, respond appropriately in a particular moment. The encounter with Mr. Jones sparked a question that I hope, at this point, never burns out. *How am I to pay attention to what all matters in this moment, which already exceeds and disorders whatever expectations I had going into it?*

In the encounter with Mr. Jones, I was completely gob-smacked. I was thrown back on myself – suddenly unsure of why I was there (and whether I should be); unexpectedly uncertain about what and how I was supposed to learn. Every part of me was a quivering antenna – all senses activated. My mind was whirling in different directions and latching onto details because everything and anything I saw, heard, smelled, felt – every movement seemed critically important. Or like it might be. And I wasn't sure I could tell anymore, or what to do with it if I could. In my embodied, visceral responses to Mr. Jones's pain, and in the eternity of silent-eyed inquiry with Dr. Wiley, I cringed into uncertainty about my very self-understanding as a student, indeed, as a person. But why the doubt?

In those moments, my focus was both directed by my curiosity and pulled by actions or objects or communication before I was aware my attention had shifted. I wasn't sure I would be able to figure out what was happening as it was happening – or even identify what might matter as things were happening. I wasn't sure if I should stay or go – or what my responsibility was and to whom. All of the things I thought I was supposed to be paying attention to and had been preparing to pay attention to swirled around and got mixed up with what I *found* myself paying attention to or being drawn into seeing. This included the suddenly sharp recognition that I was trying to pay attention to what and how I was paying attention while being attentive to all of it. A complex loop, for sure, being thrown back again and again, like being tumbled by the breakers where the ocean crashes into land.

Experiencing my attention as being drawn, rather than directed, feeling reactive rather than intentional, I was then keenly aware that my deep uncertainty and unknowing – after months of accumulated experience and knowledge – felt like a failure, a profound inadequacy. Despite preparation and intention, I found myself feeling wildly unprepared and worrying that those feelings meant my presence was illegitimate, unwarranted. I was caught by the experience of being a Stranger still, disrupted by what I was seeing, and feeling uncertain of how to pay attention to and understand the encounter, or myself in it. *All of those things that had led me to being in that moment were brought into question by that moment*: as if I was now undergoing some sort of clarification in my preparation, knowledge, and skills for watching how to interact with others, what I was seeing, and how I was understanding.

In neither the encounter with Mr. Jones nor the more mundane MICU moments, however, was I fully aware of those nuances of the experience or, able to identify and articulate them as I can now, years later. I was simply *in* that moment or set of moments while they occurred, but I recognized something powerful in the encounter. I spent the two semesters that followed trying to articulate, frame, understand, manage, and make sense of the experience of being disrupted. I wrote and interrogated myself via journals, papers, and discussions with my teachers, trying to get clear enough to continue entering the clinical setting, to keep returning to Seminar each week. And still, the encounter with Mr. Jones demanded attention and I knew I wasn't done reflecting on it or looking for a frame for understanding it. I wanted to find some way I could move past this disruption (and any others like it!) toward paying attention, being intentional in my learning.

### Encountering Kurt Wolff's Surrender-and-Catch

What I discovered, instead, was a method for thinking about the movement between disrupted attention and deliberate attention, for acknowledging both as pathways for making sense of human experiences. Midway through my clinical training and Seminar years at Vanderbilt, I was introduced to the writings of Kurt H. Wolff, an accomplished social scientist and observer, a philosopher by any other name. In a startlingly complex book, *Surrender and Catch: Experience and Inquiry Today,* published in 1976,[3] Wolff articulates the compelling experience of finding oneself "thrown back on oneself," out of what is known and taken-for-granted – and into the possibility of understanding something new instead. Wolff's "surrender-and-catch" offers a way to make sense of the broadly human experience of encountering things we may not understand, but which matter deeply to us once encountered.

Wolff describes the experience of surrender as being thrown back on oneself by an unchosen, befallen experience – and that in the five elements of surrender there emerges the possibility of a new understanding, of insights, of a catch. It is important to note here that in *Surrender and Catch*, Wolff also includes surrender-to as a deliberate approach to learning or toward understanding that makes intentional and careful use of elements of surrender to purse possible understandings. The surrender is attention drawn and unchosen, while the surrender-to is attention disciplined and deliberate – and each holds the possibility (though never the promise) of understanding. Surrender-to is a practice that allows for the stunning disruption of the surrender to become an occasion for perplexity, and curiosity, "to pay utmost attention"[4] in this sense of wanting to learn or know more about what happened.

Wolff and his work came into my world indirectly, via Richard M. Zaner's review-cum-essay, "The Disciplining of Reason's Cunning: Kurt Wolff's '*Surrender and Catch*'" published in *Human Studies* five years after Wolff's book.[5] Both Zaner's review and, later, my direct encounter with Wolff's book were challenging and enriching: the concept of surrender-and-catch both resonated and repelled, not unlike the experience with Mr. Jones in the MICU. This approach both seemed to fit in terms of what I was learning – and simultaneously was wholly unlike anything I had expected or had imagined. Both Wolff's ideas, and Zaner's explications and expansion were dense, convoluted, and disconcerting: they felt both accessible and esoteric. It took me some time and significant effort to realize that the indirections in both *Surrender And Catch* and "The Disciplining of Reason's Cunning" are deliberate and necessary. In fact, these indirections are part of a deliberate method for reflecting on the interplay of disrupted attention, controlled and focused attention, and the possibilities of understanding. These philosophical texts were deeply clinical.

The writing itself, in both the unfolding of Wolff's book and Zaner's essay, put the reader in touch with the experience of surrender – with the possibility (but not guarantee) of a catch. I struggled fiercely, sensing that there was something helpful – meaningful if I could work my way to it – but visible only obliquely, spinning just out of range just when I thought I'd figured it out. What a way to create and embody the experience being described to the reader as they are reading! And yet, what a challenge to a graduate student in the midst of multiple iterations of her own disruptive experiences, in Seminar and in the MICU, riding waves and crests and crashes of clinical experiences. I was looking for something to help me tread water. Instead, I encountered Zaner's and Wolff's offer that the drowning moments are *to be expected,* as *given,* as perhaps even *necessary* experiences. I was reluctant to take them up on these offers.

More accurately, I resisted them, and it took me years of clinical practice and continued efforts to try to account for, reflect on, and engage with others about just these sorts of disruptions to realize that Wolff and Zaner were, in the language of my religious studies background, *practicing what they were preaching.* They were showing that disrupted attention illuminates something about ongoing experience, that it's not merely a stage along the way to be mastered and moved past; that the "real work" of understanding emerges in the experience. Wolff's *Surrender And Catch* gives an account of the experience of having one's attention, and one's intention toward making sense, caught and captured, and yet which still holds the possibility of understanding something we didn't intend or to which we did not deliberately attend. The movements between certainty and disruption, knowing and unknowing, uncertainty and understanding are fits-and-starts, choppy waves. Wolff's own push/pull shifts of attention and topic in the text move his reader along with him, between the taken-for-granted ways of knowing and attending to experiences, and the novel or surprising encounter that bring learning beyond what we expect.

Years later, I read Wolff's surrender-and-catch and the surrender-to as offering a parallel to my hard-to-articulate encounter with Mr. Jones in the MICU: both the visceral disruption in his room and all that had become taken-for-granted *so quickly* in the months of diligent and dedicated attention on rounds which led up to that moment. What follows is intended to illustrate those parallels – and the elements of surrender that I found and still find so resonant to clinical ethics work.

### Elements of Wolff's Surrender

For Wolff, the initial moment of surrender is an unchosen, befallen experience of disrupted attention and intention, with five distinct elements. First, the person experiencing such disruption, the surrenderer, is thrown back on themselves, in total involvement – the experience is everything in that moment. Second, the surrender is a whole-person experience where the surrenderer finds themselves in a suspension of received notions, recognizing that previous experiences and knowledge may not be enough to make sense of the current moment or the questions at hand. Third, in the vastness of this suspension, everything seems relevant, potentially, and so brings further layers of disconcerting uncertainty of how to discover what matters. Fourth, the surrenderer finds themselves deeply invested in and concerned with what matters and so they themselves are at stake as well: it *matters to them,* and so, fifth, the potential for harm – for misunderstanding or responding wrongly – is great. The surrender is not a benign experience – which is part of why it remains an unchosen, befallen one.[6]

Yet in the wild, expansive disruption of the surrender, the possibility for new knowledge or understanding is present as a *catch.* When everything is blown open beyond expectation and imagination, beyond accepted knowledge and expected/expectant mastery, what becomes possible is unanticipated learning, unchosen insights, and novel understandings. However, Wolff is unmistakable: getting crystal clear can reveal sharp edges. The understanding in or of the catch is not an unmixed blessing: you might not like what you learn or your understanding may lead to new uncertainties or disruptions. The catch is not guaranteed; it will not necessarily resolve the uncertainty that spurred the surrender; and even if the surrenderer experiences the catch, such insights and understandings don't always redeem the disruption of the surrender. Wolff's explication of the surrender lays bare the disruption of attention, and the inability to prepare for the befallen-ness of being thrown into question without choice or intention.

### Elements of Wolff's Surrender-to

At the same time as he details the befallen-ness of surrender, Wolff explores the possibility of preparing and practicing a deliberate attention, engaging with and utilizing the elements of disrupted attention toward understanding, which he calls the *surrender-to*.[7] Wolff explores the surrender-to as the intentional pursuit of understanding the experience of a surrender. Not so much the disruption itself – since that is unchosen and befallen – but the *kinds* of attention and concern, what he attributes to cognitive love, the catch that comes into[8] the surrender and can be practiced in the surrender-to, engaged with as a discipline, as a method. Wolff's explanations help show why cognitive love becomes so relevant to clinical ethics. He notes,

> Every experience itself is a touch. Whatever or whoever it may be. Some of us have tried to understand what or who touches us, in whatever form the touch reaches us: it may be, to mention only a few, a hardly perceptible breath, or a slap, or a task of whatever kind, or love or hate in their uncountable ways, or an illness, or a change, prepared for or unexpected, in our material condition, or the happiness or the death of a beloved friend or relative, or myself.[9]

In whatever form these experiences occur, Wolff says,

> If we are aware in any way of our experience, of its touch, we may make an effort to account for it. This happens if the experience impresses us so as to raise questions about it and if the questions have no ready-made answer provided by our socialization. One response to such a situation is 'surrender.'[10]

If Mr. Jones was my experience in surrender, perhaps a catch was my growing awareness of my surrender-to: that I had been preparing for that moment long before I knew what I would be doing. The Mr. Jones encounter became a pivotal point for my recognition of and working into the concepts of surrender-to as a discipline, making an effort to account for clinical ethics practice. Wolff's surrender and the possibility of a catch frame my story of Mr. Jones as the reminder of how unexpected disruption can be – how unavoidable when it befalls. Likewise, Wolff's surrender-to frames my understanding of the ways intentional engagement with those elements of disruption can become both preparation and practice for clinical ethics work. While the Mr. Jones story remains an exemplar of surrender – and an opportunity for ongoing reflection – my training journals, notes and verbatims from my MICU rounds offer examples of how I practiced elements of surrender in the day-to-day discipline of surrender-to.

### Clinical Ethics Rounds and the Discipline of Surrender-To

The dimensions of surrender-to were already present and practiced in my clinical ethics observations, in my exposure to MICU rounds during my "Internship in Clinical Ethics" and the large volume of journals/reflective writings that came out of them. They remain available for reflection even now: *Total involvement. Surrender of received notions. Pertinence of everything. Identification. Risk of harm.* I carried all of these into the first day of rounds – even before rounds – and still.

As an example of seeing the dimensions of surrender in the practices of surrender-to: my journal entry from *before* my first day in the MICU shows clear efforts, however halting and self-conscious, to be reflective, to be wide-ranging – even comprehensive – in the topics I wanted to pursue. I wrote self-consciously, trying to identify my assumptions and pre-figured ideas, a gulping awareness of how much was at stake for me in beginning this phase of my education and training:

> *Well, this is the beginning I suppose. Odd to be writing a journal you know other people will be reading, probably very closely. Keeping this journal is one of the requirements for the Internship in Clinical Ethics, as is meeting with Drs. Finder and Bliton once a week to discuss my experiences, thoughts, and reflections on what I see and hear. We met today to discuss where I will be and what I will be doing, though I still have only a vague sense of my role at this point. I hope it will clear up once I get started on Monday, which will be when things really begin.*

> *Monday morning, Dr. Finder and I will join the medical residents for rounds in the Medical Intensive Care Unit (MICU) at Vanderbilt. The MICU will be my assignment for the first four weeks, perhaps longer (depending on how I'm doing and what I'm doing). This journal is supposed to be a place for me to record my experiences and reflect on them, and eventually some kind of paper (also reflective) is supposed to come out of this. I decided to start writing now to get some of my thoughts and impressions out before I begin. They will probably be interesting for comparison at different points in the semester and, indeed, over the next few years.*

> *The first thing is some kind of feeling of nervous anticipation. I have said for the past few years that this field – clinical ethics – is the field I want to pursue, but there remains the fact that I don't REALLY know that because I've never done clinical work in this field, or even seen clinical work done. My only experience comes through the writings and case studies and theories of others. Although I'm fairly confident that I will enjoy it and fairly confident that in time I could be good at this field, I won't know until I'm actually in there. So, there is some nervous anticipation as far as that goes.*

> *One of the other things is something Finder and Bliton brought up today in our discussions, which I hadn't really thought about. They gave me some cautionary advice about reactions from peoples (residents, patients, families, etc.) to my role as an ethics student and the possibility/probability that people would ask me how to approach cases or about the ethical issues involved. I have to run the gauntlet between saying, "Don't ask me! I'm just an ethics student and I don't know anything!" and "Well, let me tell you what I think ..." The first position jeopardizes my position and my relationship with the people there (residents, patients, families, etc.) because if I don't know anything, what I am doing there? The second is dangerous because I don't know anything about ethics consultations but what I've read and can't offer anyone advice. So, they suggested I try to ask about what the important issues are, or bring up what I think the important issues are and leave it at that until I talk to them. I hope I'll be able to do that. My first response in that kind of situation would be the "I don't know, I'm just a student" route, because I am very aware of how little I know in terms of practicalities and experiences of being seen as "an ethics person." I do have to remember, however, that I am not totally ignorant and that this is my opportunity to ask questions, to get involved, to see what different people see as the important factors in these situations.*

I knew I needed to pay attention to everything around me. Like Schutz's Stranger, I found my-self at risk as the not-known interloper, a recognition clear in the self-protective tone throughout the journal texts. I was worried that I wouldn't be able to figure out what was going on, if I couldn't pay attention to the "right" things. And yet, and *of course*, the paying attention was different in the imagining than in the actual experiences.

## Total Involvement

*Interesting, but not as interesting as I had expected. Interesting because I got to watch and listen to the residents, fellows, and attending physician; less interesting than expected be-cause there was little or no interaction with the patients or patients' families. There were reasons for this, as I found out later, but I was taken aback at first.*

*With the first two patients, the residents and fellows and Dr. Sanderson, the Attending phy-sician, stood in the hallway and talked about the patient with the door wide open into the semi-darkened room. They talked about each of them and then moved on to the next room. I was a little angry, wondering why they didn't go in and say hi, chat with the patient, ask how they were doing, something. It seemed kind of callous or detached. Eventually I real-ized that most of the patients were still sleeping or were not cognizant of what was going on. The few rooms where a patient was alert, they shut the door before beginning their review of the case.*

*On the other hand, in another case, where a man was pretty out of it (for lack of a more tech-nical term) there was no hesitation about entering the room and standing around the bedside while some probed his stomach (for what, I didn't catch. I hope my ear will become quicker as this goes on). The man twitched in pain at their touch, but didn't regain consciousness.*

*This happened a few more times in different rooms (though we didn't enter every room) and I continued to wonder about the almost total lack of patient and doctor interaction. All the communication and information was exchanged among the nurses and those doing the rounds.*

In looking back, I can recognize *what Wolff calls the total involvement* – the first element of sur-render. In those early days and weeks, I tried to keep an eye on and an ear out for acronyms, how people moved (or didn't), who talked and who didn't – who even was with the group on a given day – what roles people had on the team. I was fully in those moments, every time I was in the MICU, and even in the moments of writing my reflections or being in conversation with Mark and Stuart in our weekly debriefs.

In that total involvement in the MICU, everything was new different, or stood out in compari-son to things I thought I already knew, but turned out to be different. I knew I was supposed to be open, to be questioning everything, all I had brought with me. Months in, I can see the efforts to understand what I knew to be my biases.

## Suspension of Received Notions

*I'm interested in looking back, to see what I thought I was supposed to be observing. Appar-ently, I had some vision of the staff and patients/families talking about big "ethical dilem-mas" on a daily basis. I thought I would be observing doctor/nurse – patient/family relations and interactions, because aren't they, after all, the loci of ethical interactions and isn't that what I'm supposed to be learning about or observing? Apparently not. It's dawning on me that a) there's a lot more to being an "ethics person" of some (whatever) kind than just being called in for "big problems," and b) there's stuff going on, enough for reflection with just the staff and the hospital setup. I'm supposed to be (and find myself) watching the details.*

It wasn't until I encountered an experience different than my expectations that I realized how deeply rooted those expectations were – how tightly held my preconceived and *"received" notions* were until they were suspended by the reality of the clinical encounter. This is the second dimension of surrender, that Wolff calls the *suspension of received notions*, a kind of mundane phenomenological bracket.[11] In another example, I found myself surprised when I realized that there were few complex discussions on rounds about patients' goals, values, and preferences (what I thought of then as "what patients' want"). I was surprised, even a little bit primly shocked, to hear the doctors and nurses talk about what they would even be offering to one family or another, without asking what the patient "wanted." That's not how the ethics casebooks or study guides had presented the dilemmas that arose! The encounter itself raised questions that I hadn't known enough to imagine beforehand and couldn't even recognize until I'd been forced to put aside what I thought I knew.

### Pertinence of Everything

*One of the residents brought up concerns she'd heard from the patient's daughters about what to do next. Dr. Sanderson asked where the daughters were, if they were in the waiting room. It was the nurse's response that struck me. She said, "Wherever they're not supposed to be, that's where they usually are." This was said in a fairly caustic tone of voice, so I assume she'd had a lot to bear from the daughters, but I wonder what. Are they demanding? Do they try to tell the nurses what to do? Or are they too present and getting in the nurses' way too much? Why did the nurse sound so bitter?*

*Dr. Sanderson pointed out to the residents that the woman wasn't getting any better, that there was a risk of infections from IV lines and catheters, and that she'd like to be paged the next time the daughters arrived so she could talk to them. She said, "Being in the hospital can be really bad for your health" and pointed out that when people get old they get fragile, even things done to help them can push them over the edge. Dr. Sanderson opened the question of moving to comfort care. One resident (Dr. Hill) asked what she meant by comfort care. Dr. Sanderson replied, "It means what you want it to mean. It could mean anything." She went on to say that comfort care is always a goal, but in this case, she was referring to the withdrawal of artificial support. Dr. Sanderson also pointed out that comfort care should be directed at the family too, and suggested that the residents/fellows could take responsibility for the decision from the family by telling them that there is nothing further to be done for the woman and that continued support is prolonging death rather than saving life. She suggested having conversations with the family about whether they wanted to be in the room when the machines are slowed or turned off. She and one of the fellows also talked about ways to slow the machines (like ventilators) rather than turning them off totally or taking out the breathing tubes. In the latter case, the patient often struggles, makes "gurgling" sounds, and appears in discomfort as he or she dies. In the former, by slowing the drug and nutrient drips and the ventilators to almost nothing, the family gets a sense of a peaceful death.*

*In contrast, the other interesting patient was a Dr. Cameron, because a) he had a family member there (daughter) b) he was somewhat responsive (you had to yell loudly so he could hear, but he responded to commands) and c) he is very ill with some kinds of infection (three different microbes, I thought I heard) and is not likely to come out of this. His fever spiked at 107° (if I heard correctly) and Dr. Sanderson spoke of that as "severe neurological insult."*

*So, Dr. Cameron's daughter seemed to be somewhat familiar with the medical terminology Dr. Sanderson used, and though Dr. Sanderson was the only one who spoke to the daughter, the rest of the group was in the room as well. Dr. Sanderson spoke matter-of-factly, asked about other family members and the DNR orders. The daughter had asked that the team do all they can until her other sisters arrived and they could decide together. Dr. Sanderson gave what felt like a kind warning or notice that they might have some difficult decisions to make in the near future. I liked the fact that she spoke so kindly to the daughter and listened to the daughter's concerns. I was also happy that she gave some sort of "advanced warning" that there were some tough choices coming up. It seems (from my experience) that even if people know on some instinctive or gut-level that they need to be thinking about difficult choices, that they will avoid such thinking as long as possible. In this case, I thought Dr. Sanderson laid the matter on the table very delicately, giving the daughter some time to prepare herself for whatever decisions might come.*

*After looking back through my notes and thinking about Dr. Cameron and his daughters, I did notice something odd (maybe) about decisions in different cases. In Dr. Cameron's case, it seems like Dr. Sanderson was preparing the daughter or giving her warning that she and her sisters might have to make some difficult choices soon. In the case of the woman who was not showing much improvement, and whose family was "wherever they weren't supposed to be," it seemed like the doctors were making choices about what was available.*

*I suppose that's why it's different – in Dr. Cameron's case, the residents are still taking care of him, whereas in this other case, they are taking care of the family by removing the weight of decision from them. The residents think the family will feel guilty if the decision to "pull the plug" is their own. The doctors can do nothing else for the patient except ease her from life, but they can help the family by making the death as easy as possible. Maybe there are other reasons as well.*

*It just struck me that there was a difference in the way that Dr. Sanderson and the residents approached Dr. Cameron's family and the other woman's family in their conversations. Do the doctors get to decide when it is time for and what form comfort care will take? It seemed like they wanted to involve Dr. Cameron's family in that decision, but to "spare" the woman's family from that same decision. Why? Maybe because Dr. Cameron's daughter seems well educated and understanding of what's going on, she gets to make decisions. Maybe the woman's family are not educated and so the doctors don't want them involved in making the decision. Would Dr. Cameron's family be better able to contribute to the conversation about decisions than the woman's family? Or, are the two cases dissimilar on some other level that I am not aware of and I'm reading the whole thing wrong? I'm not sure, and by the time I get back, they might not even be there and I might not know. Maybe I can ask someone ....*

No sooner had I incorporated some activity or fact for further investigation than some new term or idea got dropped in conversation with the team, reinforcing my stranger-ness and my deep need to know. *But to know what?* In my total involvement and having to bracket received notions, I was swamped with what Wolff calls the "*pertinence of everything*" – the third dimension of surrender – trying to sort through and learn from and about everything present in the moment. On rounds, *I knew* I did not know much about what was happening, and that I needed to know more in order to understand, to be able to learn. I wrote down unfamiliar words, acronyms and abbreviations, notes about actions or conversations that I didn't understand or that seemed different than I had imagined. I bought a copy of *Gray's Anatomy* and googled definitions I didn't know, as if those would prepare me for the next days of rounds. And eventually, several weeks into the semester of rounds, I reflected on and recognized the limits of that kind of learning – that some things *weren't* pertinent in the ways I'd thought they were. And so, part of the surrender-to was becoming more intentional and attentive toward what was pertinent, what I needed to understand in a given moment, a particular experience – even the broad experience of observation rounds in general.

> *Going back over my "field notes" from rounds, I have realized I have been making notes as I go through rounds, on patients – on what is wrong with the patient, what they are trying to do in terms of treatment, whether there are any "ethical issues" at play. My notes (and let's face it, observations and reflections) look as if I've been trying to cram four years of medical education into four hours of morning rounds each week. These things do not matter to my reflections or my internship. The details of the medical problems are not my provenance at this point. The details of what is being said, who is talking, who is listening, and what tone of voice is used are what matter to my reflections. The details of intubating a coding patient are not what I should be reflecting on. Rather, the important details for me are who is the room, who answers the call, what the residents, fellows, nurses, and attendings are doing, who is cleaning up, who is talking to the patient, what the approach of the ENT doctors looked like, who was standing in the hall and what the atmosphere was like during all of this. These are the kind of things my reflections should be about and, as said before, I need to be more conscious in choosing what to observe for later reflections. My plan is to start thinking of things I want to pay attention to in the hospital and look for one or two of those every day, keeping in mind that something unexpected but important may pop up instead.*

Every detail of conversation, every interaction brought new questions, or brought old understandings into questions. The recognition that I needed to know, that the questions I encountered had become and were becoming *my* questions illustrates *identification*, the fourth element of Wolff's surrender. However, as part of a deliberate practice of surrender-to, identification required integrating and pursing my own connection to the experience in terms of what I brought into the experience, and how the experience affects me as well as the others I engaged. Looking at my journals and notes from throughout the MICU rounds, there are examples of my efforts to incorporate past experiences to make sense of the present, as well as recognitions that only came to the fore in the moments of disruption and surrender in the MICU.

*Identification*

> *Few of the residents or fellows did much to acknowledge my presence. I was introduced to Dr. Sanderson, who was welcoming, but aside from speculative glances, I didn't get much interaction with the others on the rounds – save for one slightly older male resident (fellow?) who always gestured for me to precede him through doors. I imagine some of the distance is from confusion – what I was, why I was there – as well as from my habit of not putting myself forward – something*

*I'll have to work on if I'm to get to know these people. It'll be interesting to see if and how long it will take us to get used to my presence and to form any kind of relationship.*

*Looking back again: it's interesting that I was so concerned about my "relationships" with people in the hospital when, in fact, I have yet to form any. I suppose I had some picture in my head of being in a collegial relationship with the residents – after all, we're all students, we're all about the same age, and we're all doing the same rounds. The differences, however, are too great for a relationship to develop without some effort. We're different kinds of students. They are in a student-teacher situation where they are under review and advisement, whereas I'm just watching (my review and advisement comes on Friday mornings). We're not really the same ages. I'm close in age to some of the first-year interns, but I'm still younger than all of them. And we're not doing the same rounds. Oh, we're walking the same halls, but that's where it ends. I'm listening and watching, trying to develop an ear for their conversations about patients for a variety of reasons: so I can understand the terms they use (and what they're talking about), so I can start picking out the subtexts (what's being said, not said, who's talking, who's listening) and observing what is going on among the residents, fellows, interns, nurses, other staff, and (when present) families. The residents are doing different rounds. They are talking about and making decisions on caring for these very sick people in the MICU, learning how the MICU works, how to interact with their teacher, each other, etc. We are not doing the same rounds at all. And I wonder if that fact will change at all, once I get to know them better, once I better understand what they are doing and what I am doing.*

*Yet, I'm not sure about whether there will be any kind of relationship between the other students and me. Dr. Finder and Dr. Bliton pointed out the difference between social and clinical settings. The fact that this is a "clinical" setting explains part of the interaction between the residents and me. This is not a place where someone is going to come up to the new kid and say "Hi, I'm So-and-so, who are you?" Everyone there knows his or her role and assumes that everyone else does too. I have to discover my role and participate through that role. No one's going to help me into it.*

*Which is another part of the lack of relationships. I have some pretty well ingrained inhibitions against putting myself forward in a situation where I'm not sure what's going on. Maybe I was subconsciously aware that different rules govern these interactions. Everyone in the MICU seems to know his or her "place," his or her "role" – how to act, what each other person does, etc. I'm kind of an unknown quantity as of yet – who is this ethics student and what is she doing here? And it appears that I will have to address those unasked questions by volunteering the information. No one is going to ask me why I'm there. I have to tell them: I'm an ethics student, working on a Ph.D., and I'm interested in clinical ethics consultations. I'm here to observe how the hospital works, what different people do, and what kinds of things are important in a hospital setting. I hope this is going to be the first of many levels of training and experience so that I can one day work as a clinical ethics consultant.*

*So, the next step is actually saying that to people. And following it with some form of question(s) about what I want to know. Which means I have to figure out what it is I want to know.*

My self-identification with what I was doing in those clinical rounds is striking to me now – and it continued throughout those weeks. How could I be in this group of strangers, but where I was the Stranger? How could I learn and ask and be present in ways that work within the invitation and expectations of others, many of which remain unclear to me? How much of my hesitation is personal and idiosyncratic – my own awareness of my temperamental shyness or socialized self-effacement? How much is an appropriate response to the phenomenon of being the Stranger approaching the in-group – at risk of exclusion or expulsion *and* encompassing acceptance or difference-erasing inclusion? These questions mattered *to me* in real ways and affected the shape and texture of interactions with others: they were part of the moral encounter of learning in the clinical setting.

### *The Risk of Harm*

*After everyone finished discussing x-rays, Dr. Sanderson moved them back into the hallway towards a white board and got ready to talk to them about some procedure or condition that I missed the name of. Before she started, I shook her hand, made my goodbyes, and turned to do down the hallway. She called after me and said, "Feel free to ask any questions or raise any issues you want to during rounds." I smiled and thanked her and walked back to address the group. I said, "Actually this is a good opportunity for me to kind of generally introduce myself to everyone. I'm an ethics Ph.D. student, doing rounds with you all to get a feel for what goes on in the hospital. I would love it if any of you could talk to me, at your convenience, about what it's like to be a resident, to see patients, and talk to families." I explained that I would be back on Thursday, but having missed two weeks due to illness, I was hoping to come more frequently next week. I saw several nods of "Ah ... I get it now" and several smiles of encouragement that seemed to promise willing conversationalists. And so, as hard as it was to address the group like that, especially on the spur of the moment, I felt like it was one of the most productive parts of the day and a minor victory in my steps towards talking to the residents more intimately. I also think they seemed relieved to have a better sense of who I was and what I would be doing with them.*

The identification of oneself in the experience of the surrender (and the deliberate acknowledgement and engagement with oneself in the practice of the surrender-to) allows for a kind of openness and intention in learning that I struggled to name, to engage with in the early months and even years of my clinical education. I struggled to accept and internalize that such identification and engagement is not only authorized but also expected, and that it also demanded an accounting of my experiences – before, during, and after any given encounter. The perceived threat of not-knowing extended to my own not-knowing – what if I didn't even know what I was thinking or why, or couldn't account for what I said or did, or what if my rationales and understandings weren't sufficient, or were simply *wrong*? I experienced that not-knowing as risk to my self-understanding, as painful vulnerability that I wanted to minimize, to ameliorate by focusing on whatever else was happening in the circumstances at hand.

The idea and implications of seeing myself as morally relevant, as contributing to the ethical dimensions of the encounter felt transgressive and risky. The risk was part imposter syndrome, part lingering commitment to some deep beliefs that there was an external, objective body of knowledge to be acquired, a skill set to be mastered, that would allow me to *know* and *do* this work of clinical ethics in the "right way." Despite Mark and Stuart's invitations to consider otherwise, at the time I was still committed to some imagined ideal of knowledge, procedure, outcome – and perhaps avoidant of considering my own experience as demanding inquiry.

### Surrender-to as Responsibility for Attention

Wolff's insight for surrender – which is available in the surrender-to – is that while such experiences create a risk of harm – to self as much as to potential others – it also creates possibilities for authentic understandings. In these journals, what gets revealed is the vulnerability of exposing one's unknowing and uncertainty – that the surrender and even the surrender-to force a recognition of how self-protective we are even in our attempts at learning.

*In my talk with Drs. Finder and Bliton on Friday, we discussed how I know when the residents know what they are talking about, how I know they are giving a correct answer when the fellow or attending asks a specific question. The conversation was about how I reflect on what I observe:*

*Can I bracket my pre-conceptions about the knowledge they have as residents and pick up on what else is going on?*

*Who asks the questions? Who answers? How do they answer?*

*Why that person and not this person?*

*What is this person doing while the question is asked?*

*How does the questioner acknowledge a right answer?*

*What do they do with a wrong answer?*

*What does the person who answers do when they are right? Are wrong?*

*When are the questions asked?*

*What does all of this tell me about how the residents learn?*

*What are they learning?*

*What does it say about the power structures of the teaching service? About what is happening in front of my eyes?*

*Why does it matter to me? Does it matter to anyone else but me?*

*What other questions am I not asking because of some pre-conception that I haven't noticed or bracketed?*

*These are the same kinds of questions I need to be asking about a lot of (all of?) my experiences doing rounds. It relates, I think, to the "intentionality" that Finder and Bliton stress. It gets to the questions I was asking in my last reflection entries about why I am doing what I'm doing and what I hope to get out of these rounds. What am I looking for? As I've been doing rounds these past few weeks since I've been better, I've been "getting a feel" for what goes on in the MICU. That is how I have described what I'm doing to people in the hospital and to people in my daily life who ask. Now that I am "getting a feel" for what goes on, it is time for me to start being more intentional about what I'm doing, to start bracketing my pre-conceptions about what goes on, and about what I'm doing. I sat Friday morning, trying to figure out what Dr. Bliton was after when he was asking about how I know, listening to he and Dr. Finder go back and forth about what they were really asking and realizing that I need to be participating. And I realized I need to sit down and figure out what it is that I am trying to learn in this internship. Observation and description are part of it, but reflecting on what I observe and describe, whatever it is that I observe and describe, is more important, as is consciously choosing what it is \*I\* am trying to observe and describe.*

I see even in these still early reflections the diligent efforts to structure and direct my learning, to seek out what it is I thought I should know – to manage it all. I was still committed to some imagined ideal of knowledge, "critical distance," procedure, and outcome that was entirely about other people. It is striking to think about now: what a self-protective frame that was! In reflecting on that disconnect, I wonder how much of the clinical ethics field's commitment to that kind of "critical distance" (even today!) is rooted in efforts to manage and even master the fifth element of Wolff's surrender: *the potential for harm* in the surrender and surrender-to.

The risk of harm in clinical ethics work is ever present and multivalent – and not always explicitly addressed. In recognizing the potential for harm to myself (I might be misunderstood, I may not have enough knowledge, I may be wrong), I also must acknowledge that I carry and bring with me the risk of harm to others (I may not understand them, they may need something I can't provide, I may be wrong in the ways I engage them or the type of support I offer). While trying to engage with and responsibly incorporate my own identification (through attention, reflection, accounting with and to others), I may be harming others *because* of my identification with the circumstance or some other person in the encounter. Or *with* the recognition that previously received notions are insufficient. Or *because* I am overwhelmed by the total involvement and the pertinence of everything. In pursing the questions and clarity that emerge as needed in a clinical context, I may also be opening wounds for others; poking around in skeleton-filled closets or holding up mirrors to people intentionally hiding from themselves. My presence alone – as ethics consultant – may be the spark that ignites another's surrender, unchosen and overwhelming. The potential for harm – from the threats of unknowing and disruption perceived and experienced as harm – is inherent in the work. Awareness of it is one of the striking elements of the experience of surrender, and the deliberate practice of the surrender-to: one that must be identified, attended to, faced, even embraced as morally relevant and ethically significant in what all matters.

### The Particular Matters for Responsible Practice

As I wrote in December of that first year of rounds, the disruption of the moment and experience of surrender with Mr. Jones, was as much about me – my learning, my experience, my understanding – as a relevant factor in the clinical encounter, as anything else. That in itself brought to attention my own moral engagement in a deeply disconcerting way. *Recognizing that my individuated experience had relevance to and connection to something that is deeply human and broadly present – and as such deserved and required attention alongside the experiences of the Others in the encounter felt transgressive and risky. There was not a case book for that disconcerting realization.* My MICU journals bear witness:

> *What was I supposed to do in this observation, pushing aside for the moment whether I was "supposed" to be there in the first place? As the family and PharmD students and librarian filed out the room, these questions flickered in and out of my head, along with the thought that perhaps I needed to be there. Not for the patient, not for the housestaff, but that I needed to be there and I needed to see what was happening for me.*

> *Why? When I first decided to do this internship, I wanted to get practical experience in the hospital, to see what happens, and see what it was like to be an "ethics person" among patients, nurses, doctors, and other staff. I knew that, though I have wanted to do clinical ethics for years, I still did not really know what that meant. I didn't know if I could do it. I didn't know if I could handle it. I wasn't even sure what "it" was, and I knew that I needed some "hands-on" experience before I could address any of those questions. Underlying all of this*

*was a question, a fear almost of what if, after deciding on medical ethics as my career and scholarly goal, I come to find out that I hate it, or I'm not good at it? I decided I should jump into this internship as soon as possible to discover if I wanted to jump right back out or not.*

The encounter with Mr. Jones – and all that it raised in terms of disruption and vulnerability – persists as the catch of my earliest clinical training in that it remains available as a source for self-reflection and engagement with others. It is something I carry with me – not because it's something I can't put down or get past, but because *that* surrender-and-catch is an experience that shapes the other experiences that followed: from shortly after two years later, clinical encounters are often disruptive, and fertile, and available for self-reflection. My deepest learning of that early training was something I could not have chosen, nor prepared for before the encounter. It was the encounter itself that carried its own fragile, accidental, never-guaranteed possibility for understanding: for me to discover what and how I could learn, from within my own need to understand.

### Practicing Surrender-to: An Invitation to Reflective Clinical Ethics

Another disruptive thought ends these reflections on the disruptive and iterative elements of undergoing surrender in clinical ethics work: I might never have had the moment of openness and learning of surrender-and-catch. The encounter with Mr. Jones might not have generated reflection and development of new questions from that disruption. The surrender-and-catch and moments of moral experience are not chosen. They come unbidden and *befall* us, as Wolff insists. But often, and in this encounter, the surrender would not have happened without the build-up of training and preparation from Seminar on through early rounds. The surrender-to practice of using the tools, "recipes," patterns and habits already developed was necessary to investigate and interrogate the concerns at hand, even if I couldn't see at the time that was what I'd been doing. The Mr. Jones story stands out as an example of disruption of attention that emerged along with and after all the preparation and efforts to manage my attention and learning.

So much of the work in the field and so many of the trainings and processes seem to focus on the analysis and the management of disruption: if we can get things in the right categories, we won't experience them as disruptive. Or we'll constrain and contain the disruption, make sure it wipes its feet at the door and maintains appropriate decorum. We won't get lost in it. In more recent iterations of our field, many seem to have added further the idea that if we can point to something and say "this is quality" then we'll none of us be disrupted by the kind of wondering that comes, unbidden and uncontrolled, from this work.

Perhaps in a more typical "How to Become a ..." book, I would be explaining that the Mr. Jones encounter was the first time I felt so overwhelmed and flabbergasted but that with practice and helpful tools I learned to overcome or avoid these types of experience. As you might now imagine, Mr. Jones stays with me because I have had this kind of experience in so many contexts that I no longer keep count. The recurrence and persistence of these kinds of experiences form a bright tenuous thread I continue to unspool in each clinical encounter: can I learn from and with these people what matters for them? In this moment? Can I learn how I learn whatever it is and understand my own learning? For them, for me, for the next one? In each consult, remembering I am here to learn and to model and embody and engage that learning – because maybe the others are in their own surrender – unchosen, unavoidable, despite the defenses and management and efforts at control, their intentions and the preparations of the surrender-to ....

Wolff's opening acknowledgment that the surrender is something that *befalls* the surrenderer – unbidden, unchosen, in some ways unmanageable – is deeply relevant for and crucial for clinical ethics work. The possibility of being disrupted, of being thrown back on oneself, despite whatever preparation and training one has, is ever present in each clinical encounter – for any and all of the participants, ethics consultant included. I am not arguing that every clinical encounter or engagement as a clinical ethics consultant will necessarily be or even accidently be a gob-smacking, overwhelming, possibly enlightening moment of disruption and surrender or surrender-and-catch. But I am asserting that such a possibility is part of the moral landscape of engaging with people in *their* crisis of illness, injury, or caring for those who are ill or injured.

What Wolff's work does, then, is offers a way to make sense of such disruptive experiences of *not* understanding and *needing* to understand as to-be-expected in clinical ethics consultation. The surrender is not something to be avoided or managed but recognized and learned from in each encounter. Wolff's work offers a frame for understanding experiences of disruption caused by encountering something that you are compelled to understand, that matters deeply. The surrender-to allows for the conscientious interrogation of one's own practices, tools, recipes, patterns, and habits – at least to a certain degree. Surrender – especially if it becomes a surrender-and-catch, carries the possibility (both promise and threat) of encountering and discovering things you could not even question because they were so deeply embedded, so tied to identity and self. But because they are put into question by an encounter with *Someone Other* or *Other People*, there is the emergence of, the possibility of the catch. In these encounters, we may find an understanding that can be shared with *Some Other* or *Some Others*, to connect and reflect and corroborate and challenge further. To surrender, again, together.

## Notes

1  Schutz, Alfred (1944). The stranger: An essay in social psychology. *American Journal of Sociology* 49 (6):499–507.
2  *Grosse Pointe Blank* (1997). Directed by George Armitage. Written by Tom Jankiewicz, D.V. DeVincentis, Steve Pink, and John Cusack. Burbank, CA: Buena Vista Pictures, 107 min.
3  Wolff, Kurt H. (1976). Surrender and Catch: Experience and Inquiry Today. *Boston Studies in the Philosophy and History of Science*, vol. 51. Dordrecht: Springer.
4  Wolff, *Surrender and Catch*, 25–26.
5  Zaner, Richard M. (1981). The disciplining of reason's cunning: Kurt Wolff's '*Surrender and Catch*'. *Human Studies* 4 (4):365–389.
6  Wolff, *Surrender-and-Catch*, 20–26.
7  *Ibid.* 25–26; 59.
8  The sexually charged language in Wolff's text is meant to convey generative intent – see discussion *Surrender and Catch*, 20–21.
9  Wolff, Kurt H. (2003). Writing my approach to the world. *Human Studies* 26:293–308, p. 301.
10 *Ibid.*
11 Wolff, Kurt H. (1984). *Surrender-and-Catch* and phenomenology. *Human Studies* 7:191–210, p. 193.

## Bibliography

*Grosse Pointe Blank* (1997). Directed by Armitage, George. Written by Tom Jankiewicz, D.V. DeVincentis, Steve Pink, and John Cusack. Burbank, CA: Buena Vista Pictures, 107 min.

Schutz, Alfred (1944). The stranger: An essay in social psychology. *American Journal of Sociology* 49 (6):499–507.

Wolff, Kurt H. (1984). *Surrender-and-catch* and phenomenology. *Human Studies* 7:191–210.

Wolff, Kurt H. (2003). Writing my approach to the world. *Human Studies* 26:293–308.

Wolff, Kurt H. (1976). Surrender and Catch: Experience and Inquiry Today. *Boston Studies in the Philosophy and History of Science*, vol. 51. Dordrecht: Springer.

Zaner, Richard M. (1981). The disciplining of reason's cunning: Kurt Wolff's '*Surrender and Catch*'. *Human Studies* 4 (4):365–389.

# Interlude I: Methods for Unknowing
## Disruption and Attention

Seminar and Mr. Jones in the MICU. Schutz and Wolff. Both the encounters and the thinkers point to constitutive elements of clinical ethics practice – disruption and attention, specifically, the stranger's disruption and the attentional focus of the surrender-and-catch. Disruption and surrender-and-catch are both unchosen experiences, perhaps shared in different ways by an ethicist and those they are trying to help in clinical ethics work. That combination also makes them deliberate practices for those engaging in clinical ethics work.

### The Orientation of the Stranger

On my first readings of Schutz, I got caught by the role of the Stranger – the outsider-ness; the experience of disruption and not-knowing. What it felt like to be uncertain, alone, in unfamiliar territory. The radical differences of the strange land and the approached group, complicated by the subtle variations, which are perhaps more disconcerting in their uncanny, not-quite-right-ness, emerging as potentially threatening to the stranger's known and taken-for-granted recipes for living. These ideas resonated deeply with my experiences in, and my thinking about, the disconcerting newness, the *unfamiliar* circulating through that familiarity of Seminar and of MICU rounds. However, over time, and with concentrated reflection, what stands out about the stranger is less the disruption, and more about the activities and orientations the stranger deploys, engages in, and works through in the disruption of not-knowing – on the way to making sense of and finding meaning, to perhaps even understanding the differences that seem so disruptive.

The stranger's activities include hyperattentive awareness of what is similar or different from the old country; what language and which meanings map word-for-word, and which require halting and tentative translations from the mother-tongue. The stranger's method includes careful questioning to check meanings and misunderstandings, to get clear on motives and possibilities for actions; testing the situation to determine: is this a topic about which my general understanding will suffice?[1] Where do my taken-for-granted stocks of knowledge sufficiently overlap with these others? Or do the differences encountered with these other people need investigation and exploration, more discussion and discovery? The stranger's orientation is one of weird hope, perhaps unjustifiable, that understanding is possible,[2] especially in circumstances where it is desperately needed in the approach to a new community or situation. After all, it is no small thing to find oneself out of the familiar and the known, uncertain about the presumed safety of one's taken for granted "provinces of meaning" and communities.[3] The stranger is drawn to, perhaps startled and overwhelmed with the acute and immediate differences, looking for and hoping to find points of connection and similarity, even if not typical familiarity. The sharp observations, searching through the onslaught of newness, are what the stranger uses to navigate, trying to at least keep the conversation going.

DOI: 10.4324/9781003354864-5

What Schutz offers regarding a method or model for clinical ethics practice is the relevance of a stranger's awareness of their own difference and strangeness in two significant ways. First, the stranger's awareness of their strangeness serves to orient or provide a location from which to explore, interrogate, evaluate, and act in relation to the others encountered. Awareness of one's own outsider status and experience brings both the familiar and strange into sharp relief and can thus focus attention on the range of choices and the circumstances in which action is needed. The second point about this orientation and its relevance to method is more challenging: the stranger's awareness of their own strangeness and the disruption undergone in that strangeness can focus attention toward and open awareness with others who may disrupted as well, even those within the supposed "in-group" or the approached context.

This latter is a particularly potent activity, especially in the realm of clinical ethics consultation because it runs counter to the dominant, even totalizing rationalities of the field: philosophical and biomedical, economic and political. The stranger's hypervigilance in the face of disruption and uncertainty offers a reminder that the clinical ethics consultant cannot be at ease in their inquiry and attention: no matter the ready appeal of proceduralism and principlism. The method, then, acknowledges that each clinical encounter can reveal its own strange new world, and present its own *sui generis* interaction for everyone involved, and so demands the attention, careful questioning, and constant reflexivity encountered in being a stranger. Even further, due to the dynamic character of clinical situations, each clinical encounter carries the unavoidable possibility of the stranger's disruption evolving into the full, befallen overwhelm of surrender.

### The Problematic of Disruption

While the reflexivity demanded by the encounter with others opens the possibility of recognizing and responding to another's disruption, it also raises the haunting problem of those experiences and aspects in the disruption dominating the encounter; and the subsequent unchosen, unmanageable, surrender. What if none of us escape this disruption? What if we stay surrendered? What if our accumulated stocks of knowledge and recipes for acting in the world remain inadequate to realize change for our current unknowing? What if we can't find a way through this experience? The possibility of the surrender, the unexpected encounter with a disruptive, perhaps hazardous unknowing, persists until the stranger is fully acclimated and assimilated into the new group and new situation. So, the concern is not merely about whether or not becoming fully acclimated to the structures that influence clinical ethics, i.e., conceptual and empirical, may ever happen; perhaps the deeper, more unsettling question is that it should not.

In that light, there are challenges to the role of the stranger as an appropriate model, or the extent to which the stranger's activities could serve as a model for clinical ethics work, especially with this focus on the ongoing disruption and requirement for constant vigilance. One particularly helpful discussion emerged over breakfast in Singapore, at the International Conference on Clinical Ethics Consultation (ICCEC, 2017). I had organized a panel discussion about Schutz and the Stranger with my teachers and colleagues, Mark Bliton and Stuart Finder and we were most grateful to have our friend and colleague, Dr. Stella Reiter-Theil there to moderate. Stella guided a lively discussion and, as good friends and colleagues do, helped us to consider some different implications about our work and commitments by raising two challenges for us to consider.

First was the concern that the stranger's disruption – in the context of clinical ethics consultation – might weaken or limit the ethics consultant's ability to recognize and respond to the others as strangers. Specifically, Stella wondered whether the clinical ethics consultant, *as stranger* within the reflexive confines of their own disruption, could maintain an approach of openness and hospitality, of invitation and inquiry to those others – patients and families – who are themselves accidental strangers within a clinical setting. She raised the alternative idea of the ethics consultant as occupying a strange role between those coming from a "home" (non-clinical) environment to a place of "work" (a clinical environment): not to act as or engage in the role *as a stranger* with their own disruption, but to situate and ground one's practice in a *role*, in attempts to manage the danger and disruption of the stranger's experience. Stella pointed out that not every encounter is disruptive, after all, and offered a German word to consider instead of stranger: *grenzgänger* which means "border-walker" or "border-crosser." The word refers to the many who live on one side of the German-Swiss border and who work on the other, traversing regularly the boundaries between "home" and "work," between roles and identities, and familiar, although different, neighborhoods. She offered this as perhaps a more apt conception for clinical ethics than the stranger, with all the implications of danger and distance, of difference, otherness and unknowing that our panel had outlined, and which were explained in more detail in Chapter 1 on Seminar and Schutz. Professor Reiter-Theil seemed to suggest, with the idea of clinical ethicist as border-walker, that there is a sense of regularity, of routines, of recognizability as they move between different contexts.

The appeal of this idea of a boarder-walker's known, recognizable boundaries and established processes for traversing them is considerable. It holds the idea of an encounter with difference as *manageable*. It contains the wildness of the frontiers of difference and disruption. What the role of stranger carries as an advantage over the role as border-walker, however, are the attentiveness and responsiveness that are constituent within the disruption. Even with their carefulness of probing observations and deliberate, delicate questioning of points of contact, connection, and difference, the stranger cannot fully shake the distress, the discomfort of unknowing, of not being sure if they have understood, if they know where to go from here and how. The border-walker, in contrast, knows the paths and the checkpoints, the questions to be asked and answered, the documentation required to proceed. Indeed, those match up with the assumptions about a competent ethics consultant, and so that analogy sounds like the ideal approach for clinical ethics consultation practices committed to proceduralism and standardization. The problem is that this approach also reveals a disconnect from many experiences in clinical practice that the stranger highlights: not everyone knows that the procedures and actual questions may not be known or understood – by those doing the asking or those expected to answer.

The proper pathways to proceed may not be marked at all – and this is not simply for the patients and families for whom Stella was rightly concerned, but also for the clinicians and staff for whom the routine and regularized is suddenly, perhaps unexpectedly, insufficient. Political, economic, social, or other bureaucratic forces can shut down access to the roadways and leave people stranded or scrambling to find alternate pathways. The border-walker does not escape the possibility of being thrown or disrupted. Similarity and regularity do not guarantee safety or consistency. Nor, for that matter, do the Stranger's orientations and activities, and so the vigilance and vulnerability continue. The Stranger's intentional vigilance and focused attention to difference creates and allows for a responsive response to whatever disruptions emerge, yet even with the most careful method and deliberate approach to the disruption of difference and strangeness, the specter of surrender still haunts: what if we can't get out? Especially in clinical ethics practice: what if we can't get away from the disruptions or through the encounters with those we have professed to help?

## From the Stranger's Strategies to the Surrender-to

The anxiety about the overwhelm of disruption and strangeness is where Schutz's stranger connects with Wolff's surrender-and-and catch and surrender-to.[4] Schutz is quite clear that for the common sense thinking of everyday life, we assume that there is some kind of order in nature and society, yet, at root, the essence of this order is unknowable.[5] And, that limitation, that these orders in the world are rooted in elements never to be fully comprehended, is thus an inescapable feature of common sense shared by both a stranger and others. Likewise, Wolff acknowledges that, yes, we may indeed find ourselves overwhelmed by the situation at hand – disrupted and thrown by the experience that befalls us without warning, despite our preparations and intentions, perhaps even because of where our preparations and intentions have brought us. Wolff is explicit: in the moments of surrender, the surrenderer has no guarantee of emerging from the overwhelm – period – let alone with anything to learn from it, with any new knowledge or understanding. There is no assurance of being at ease ever again in the midst finding oneself unmoored by the disconnects from *before*, the strangeness of *now*, and the uncertainty of *next*. So, despite the concern Stella raised about the ethics consultant being so unsettled, it is that very experience which creates the possibility for connection and understanding between the clinical ethics consultants and the people requesting and participating in the activities of clinical ethics consultation. After all, the patients, families, and clinicians all come with their own taken-for-granted recipes for making sense of the world, their orientations and practices of "philosophizing still"[6] as their daily lives intersect with clinical contexts. The ethics consultant's experience with the stranger's disruption and experiences of the surrender-and-catch ground the possibility for both connecting to those currently surrendered strangers in a strange land *and* of modeling for them the possibility of emerging with a catch.

Wolff's surrender-to offers an approach, a method for practice because each of the aspects of surrender, of overwhelm, can be pursued in moments outside of the surrender and in dialogue, through conversation and reflective engagement, as a way to help make sense of, perhaps find meaning in the catch. Each aspect can form components for a deliberate method of working through unknowing – not unlike the deliberate and careful activities of the stranger as they engage further and more deeply with the approached group. What Wolff calls the historic and biographical can be the site – the location – for the ethics consultant and for others involved in the consultation – for connecting with the human and communal or social, both during the consultation and in its aftermath.

The practice of surrender-to offers a method to engage with the potential and actual disquiet of the stranger. Working through the features of Wolff's surrender and surrender-to (what they look like, together with what they feel like) shows that when there are still the tethers of self-reflection and self-awareness holding together, a person may be able to make some assessment and get an analyzing hook into the situation. That practice seems to make the actual moments easier to bear, whether the experiential elements of surrender come singly or in small batches, or when they approach like tsunamis, gathering strength by pulling from everything around. The moments of daily routine *and* disruptive experience become opportunities for deliberate practices and questions *for the ethics consultant* approaching clinical contexts.

As such, the elements of surrender, framed as specific questions and leaned into with deliberate care, can build into an intentional habit of surrender-to – a careful method. For example, I can ask myself: can I be fully present in this moment – without looking at watches or wondering about the next problem or project? Can I free myself from mundane concerns to be open in total involvement? Oh yes! My attention may be pulled in other directions, but I can begin with deep focus and intention to remain present, embodying the first element of surrender.

In the circumstances of a clinical ethics encounter, I can ask myself to identify my preconceived notions, my received wisdom – even about how I understand. I can reflect and consider: is this a situation, a scenario, a moral moment that fits with previous experiences? Is there something in this moment that shows, reveals what is most crucial here, now, for these people? Sometimes the assumptions and routines are all that are needed; sometimes previous tools might obscure what is most relevant – the trick is to avoid carrying hammers and seeing nails everywhere. In the surrender-to, I can actively suspend the received notions (the ones I am aware of, anyway) that would be called into question by the experience of surrender.

In suspending received notions within a deliberate effort of surrender-to, I can practice identifying and interrogating: What are the things I don't understand? How can I get clear about what I don't know and need to know? What is relevant? Can I scan the room, the chart, the communication, the personalities and see what, of all the things, needs attention? While the moments of surrender may be evoked by newness of a situation, brought on by a nearly incomprehensible amount of sensory input, not every new or disruptive experience befalls as surrender. As a practice, as method, the question becomes whether I can recognize and process the moments with the surrender-to: can I both acknowledge the potential relevances afforded by everything and begin to sort through what may be actually relevant in this particular moment?

Sorting through what may be relevant feeds further into the translation of that disruption manifest in surrender into the attention and intention of the surrender-to. Surrender contains the disruptive experience of becoming fully with the moment, while the surrender-to allows for the creation of a moral architecture, construction of intentional space.[7] Identifying myself with the moment both allows for and requires a rigorous questioning myself: can I recognize how I might be identifying with the moment in ways that may be constructive or detrimental? Am I affiliating with the others involved? Walking with someone in need? Is the fact that it is *me*, that *I* am the one in the room, something that helps another person? That I am female? A mother? Middle aged? Do the biographical facts give me insight that my non-parent colleague may not have? Or does my (contextually relative) age/youth or gender mean my older and male colleague would be more helpful, given cultural or religious commitments (or even patriarchal/systemic misogyny) of others involved? Or more concerning: can I recognize, account for, and respond to ways that my involvement may be more harmful – to them or to me? In the discipline of the surrender-to, I can be deliberately responsible for my responses to the moral encounters with others.

Since part of the disruption of the surrender is the unavoidable recognition of harm (present or potential, real or perceived), the practice of the surrender-to requires attention to the possibility of harm. The practice of surrender-to in clinical ethics work requires acknowledging that even the most careful, disciplined, best-intentioned efforts to help may still cause harm. This awareness is not intended to be paralyzing – but to elicit attentiveness, caution, and humility. It is to take seriously and find ways to avoid, mitigate, or ameliorate the harms that I might cause, especially since others may be even less able to or inclined to acknowledge such risks and harms. I recall speaking once with a colleague in palliative care medicine about a case where we had both been consulted. Their response to my query about talking with the family that afternoon was, "Sure! No big deal! Ethics is always a help!" I cringed inside, knowing that while they meant it as a compliment their enthusiasm revealed that they might not have any idea what we do or how we work. After all, the potential harm of actually probing what matters most to people at moments when it is most tender and exposed is searingly real, and points to the power of Wolff's ideas for clinical ethics practice. The fact that others may not recognize the potential for harm in clinical ethics practice only makes sharper the ethics consultant's responsibility for attending to such harms.

### Surrender as Method: A Not Entirely Benign Procedure

As part of method, the surrender-to takes seriously the pain, confusion, uncertainty, disruption, overwhelm of people confronting illness and injury, which requires acknowledging that this moment, this encounter is *new* for them *and* for the ethics consultant *and* it may be an experience of surrender for anyone involved, even, or perhaps especially, if they have "seen this before" from other experiences. In the surrender-to, deliberate attentiveness to the possibility of harm from the ethics consultant's involvement *stems from* the clinical ethics consultant's experiences of inescapable attentiveness *in a surrender* to the possibility of – or even experience of – harm, of perceived or real threat.

Asking people what matters most to them, in moments where what matters is most at issue, is serious business indeed. Doing so deliberately, intentionally, requires a willingness to face the potential for causing harm – or experiencing harm – with those already experiencing their own illness or injury. As such, the discipline of the surrender-to requires a kind of careful mutuality, and awareness of interpersonal vulnerability. Finding one's own views and commitments at stake, identified with a question or concern evoked by a given situation; unsure now about of the relevance of particular elements or even one's received notions and past experiences; being wholly involved because of a deep need to understand: these experiences are neither morally neutral nor static. The practice of the surrender-to and the encounter of surrender both open the possibility of harm that may be specific to or experienced only by the ethics consultant, at any moment, regardless of education and training, years of experience, or personal temperament. The weight of disruption, the potential for being thrown back on yourself, and the need for careful attention must be taken seriously as a relevant facet of moral encounters, especially if one is to claim recognition of and concern that the patients, families, and clinicians involved are overwhelmed, possibly surrendered, in their clinical circumstances.

For the practice of clinical ethics consultation, the challenge offered by Wolff's framework of surrender, surrender-to, and surrender-and-catch is not to stifle or contain the dimensions of total involvement, interrogation of received notions, pertinence of everything, identification and potential for harm by discounting them when they emerge from the experience of the clinical ethics consultant. After all, the dimensions of surrender are part of the experience of the patients, families, and clinicians engaging with illness and injury in healthcare settings, and as such, are part of the concern, preparation, even compulsion, that beckons to this work in the first place. Being able to articulate the dimensions of experience and practice, speak to them, share what is learned, what is broadly, humanly, relevant in the individual, historical experience – is the opportunity of the surrender-and-catch. Both Wolff's experience of surrender and the discipline of the surrender-to ask that we remain open to the possibility of learning about and discovering something *other* in the encounter with the other person, or other people in our clinical ethics practice. As the stranger, recognizing the strangeness of other people around us, we engage with them in the hopes of learning something about them, with them, maybe even understanding together. This hope and possibility points, then, to other elements of clinical ethics practice: self-reflection and self-education, along with attunement and affiliation.

## Notes

1  Schutz, Alfred (1970). *Reflections on the Problem of Relevance*. New Haven: Yale University Press.
2  James, William (1975). *Pragmatism*. Cambridge, MA: Harvard University Press; Natanson, Maurice (1962). Introduction. In Maurice Natanson (ed.), *Collected Papers of Alfred Schutz: The Problem of Social Reality*, vol. 1. The Hague: Martinus Nijhoff. pp. XXV–XLVII.
3  Schutz, Alfred (1962). On Multiple Realities. In Maurice Natanson (ed.), *Collected Papers of Alfred Schutz: The Problem of Social Reality*, vol. 1. The Hague: Martinus Nijhoff. pp. 207–259.
4  Wolff, Kurt H. (1976). Surrender and Catch: Experience and Inquiry Today. In *Boston Studies in the Philosophy and History of Science*, vol. 51. Dordrecht: Springer.

5 Schutz, Alfred (1967). Symbol, Reality, and Society. In *Collected Papers, Volume I, The Problem of Social Reality*. The Hague: Martinus Nijhoff. p. 331.
6 Bartlett, Virginia L. and Bliton, Mark J. (2022). Philosophizing still: A brief reintroduction to clinical philosophy. *American Journal of Bioethics* 22 (12):43–46.
7 Walker, Margaret Urban (1993). Keeping moral space open new images of ethics consulting. *Hastings Center Report* 23 (2):33–40.

## Bibliography

Bartlett, Virginia L. and Bliton, Mark J. (2022). Philosophizing still: A brief reintroduction to clinical philosophy. *American Journal of Bioethics* 22 (12):43–46.
James, William (1975). *Pragmatism*. Cambridge, MA: Harvard University Press.
Natanson, Maurice (1962). Introduction. In Maurice Natanson (ed.), *Collected Papers of Alfred Schutz: The Problem of Social Reality*, vol. 1. The Hague: Martinus Nijhoff. pp. XXV–XLVII.
Schutz, Alfred (1962). On Multiple Realities. In Maurice Natanson (ed.), *Collected Papers of Alfred Schutz: The Problem of Social Reality*, vol. 1. The Hague: Martinus Nijhoff. pp. 207–259.
Schutz, Alfred. (1967). Symbol, Reality, and Society. In *Collected Papers, Volume I, The Problem of Social Reality*. The Hague: Martinus Nijhoff.
Schutz, Alfred (1970). *Reflections on the Problem of Relevance*. New Haven: Yale University Press.
Walker, Margaret Urban (1993). Keeping moral space open new images of ethics consulting. *Hastings Center Report* 23 (2):33–40.
Wolff, Kurt H. (1976). Surrender and Catch: Experience and Inquiry Today. In *Boston Studies in the Philosophy and History of Science*, vol. 51. Dordrecht: Springer.

# Part II
# Elements of Learning

# 3 Self-Reflection and Self-Education in Clinical Ethics

**Unexpected Invitations in the Neonatal ICU**

"I hope it didn't sound like we don't want him or love him. You know, just because he's so sick, just because Avery isn't a perfect or a healthy baby. I'm a Christian, you know. Avery is exactly how God meant him to be and he is my perfect baby. He's not an accident, not a mistake. Do you understand? Do you have children?"

I had stopped to thank the Boones for letting me be a part of their son's care conference in the Neonatal Intensive Care Unit. My head ached and my shoulders burned from holding an attentive posture throughout the 90-minute meeting. I wanted to melt away like the residents who had slipped out after pushing in their chairs – business as usual and back to their regularly scheduled programming of taking care of sick babies. Having no routine for this moment, I defaulted to the bone-deep norms of my upbringing: leave-taking and thanks-giving required as a well-intentioned and heartfelt social nicety.

I was unprepared for being pinned to the spot by her shining, shimmering eyes, so intently focused on my face, looking for ... what? A response, I knew but what kind? Reassurance? Commiseration? Sympathy?

"No, Mrs. Boone. I don't have children, though I hope to one day." My reply was soft and awkward – muting the internal cringing. Was that too much information? A plain "No" felt harsh, but this conversation wasn't about me: I didn't want to overshare. She didn't seem to care, or even hear, really. So, my response seemed to suffice as she nodded and pressed forward:

"When you have a child, you have all these dreams that he'll be healthy – because you wouldn't have an unhealthy baby! And he'll be strong and smart and the bright point in the room and all these things." The shimmer got deeper, her voice a shattering windowpane: "When you're confronted with the realities of a sick baby, your dreams start to get smaller. My dream now for Avery is for him to breathe. Dr. Carver says he can see Avery riding a tricycle, but I can't see that far. All I can dream about is him breathing."

Her pause was longer now: looking for something this time. My words came tumbling out, as if I knew what I was talking about, knew what to say. I didn't at all, even though I meant every word:

"I understand. I can see how much you love Avery. And how hard this is. And I am so grateful to you and Mr. Boone for letting me be in the conference because I this is what I'm trying to do – to learn to understand. I am trying to figure out what matters to people, what things are important to them in moments like this ..." I paused, my eyes scanning hers this time, looking for a connection. "In my experience, most often the hopes and dreams of the families and the staff are the same. Dr. Carver can see Avery riding a tricycle and your vision may only see as far as him breathing, that you are both looking down the same path, together. That's what I've seen."

DOI: 10.4324/9781003354864-7

She took a breath and nodded sharply, as if something in what I said landed where it was needed. Or perhaps she was done with seeking validation from a stranger – from me. "Yes, I think so too," was all she replied as she began to look for her husband, still talking with Dr. Carver. They walked toward us, and I thanked Dr. Carver for inviting me, and said I would plan to see them on Wednesday for morning rounds.

I left the unit, finally, each footstep a dragging sledgehammer. The conference lasted almost an hour and a half: the combined efforts of being hyperattentive and holding myself as invisible as possible were emotionally draining and physically exhausting. What must it have been like for the others? The team? I had wanted to stay after to talk to the resident or intern – who were listening hard for the medical details while watching their attending physician model how to have such discussions. But they were gone – and on their way out the door, they hadn't looked nearly as stretched as I felt. I wanted to know their secret, to ask how and why they seemed so unfazed by the depth and breadth and the weight of that conference. But I couldn't track them down in the unit, couldn't go find them to ask. I had no space after occupying that strange corner of being present and backgrounding myself. I felt a need to get things in order in my head before I could ask any questions of the others who were present – to get away without looking like I was running away. Yet I couldn't just leave. Not without feeling rude – even if no one had really noticed or was concerned about my being there, or leaving … Dr. Carver had invited me, and the Boone's had acknowledged permission for me to observe – and those required acknowledgment and gratitude. After all, I was raised right.

And then Mrs. Boone cracked open a bit – caught in the moment of her uncertainty and her need, I found myself unsure of where – and how – to go on from there.

## Not a Solo-Sport: Clinical Self-Reflections and Self-Education with Others

After "finishing" my semester of rounds in the Medical ICU, I continued my clinical ethics training in the Neonatal ICU – this time with Mark Bliton as my primary guide and conversation partner. My experiences in the NICU were both similar to and different from MICU – and my reflections and learning were similar and wildly different as well. Mark brought me into the NICU and rounded with me frequently throughout the semester. I continued to meet with both Stuart and Mark for our Friday morning post-round debriefs, after I'd sent them my clinical journals on Thursday night, overflowing with my experiences, memories, questions, and reflections.

When Mark joined for rounds, he and I would often take time after to talk about and share the morning's observations after swinging by the coffee cart down in the hospital cafeteria and walking through the main campus. Caffeination, rumination, and perambulation. These conversations – reflecting with my teacher about my experiences – turned out to be crucial for my developing practice and my recognition of self-reflection *with others* as an important element of clinical ethics work.

I found myself building on my MICU experiences of observing, writing, and reflecting – however, one new change was that while rounding in the NICU I did more reflecting *on* my reflections in those journals and conversations. Not just the *what* of the clinical exposures but also working on *why* some things stand out more than others? *Where* did I struggle to understand? *How* was I making sense of what I encountered?

I also found that in order to talk about these encounters and experiences with others I had to be able to articulate my observations, to account for my understandings or questions – whether the discussions were with Mark on our walks, or with Stuart in the Seminar room, with the clinicians in and after rounds, or with Mrs. Boone after the care conference. I had to not only listen to and account for others' perspectives, but also to identify and reflect on my own perspectives as part of my learning and practice. In a wide variety of conversations (including the process and practice of writing and submitting my clinical journals), my teachers and the clinicians and families I encountered were helping me get clear about what was going on, how I was learning, and what all mattered in my experiences with the NICU.

At the time, I had some recognition that I was relying heavily on those around me to be able to reflect and learn – that any moments of insight and clarity I had occurred with and emerged from conversations with others. My growing understandings of the clinical context weren't things I picked up from books or that fit within a box, already mapped out: "here there be ethics!" Like other elements of clinical ethics practice, sorting out just how and why things mattered and what I was doing got clearer in revisiting those experiences. Specifically, approaching one's own moral engagement requires a kind of rigor and openness to critiques and questions from others.

Two thinkers in particular model such approaches and have become resources for considering the elements of self-reflection and self-education. First, Andrea Frolic, an anthropologist and clinical ethicist working in Canada, offers the idea of mindful embodiment as a clinical practice – and hers is a sharp critique of clinical ethics work that *doesn't* include rigorous self-reflection as part of the ethical dynamics. Second, Harald Ofstad, a Norwegian philosopher, works through the distinctions between growth and education in moral development which, although not written toward or for clinical ethics, nonetheless resonates with my understanding that while the self is crucial to moral experience, reflection and education require community: that none of us can go it alone, even (especially?) when the self is the subject at hand.

In what follows, I will look back on NICU journals using critical perspectives gained from both Frolic and Ofstad, which help illuminate the experiences and reflections on the in-the-moment encounters captured in the text of my NICU journals – and help ground the *self* part of self-reflection and self-education in communities and conversations.

### Reflecting on NICU Journals and the Practice of Self-Reflection

I keep a printout of Walt Whitman's *Leaves of Grass* above my desk, secured to the corkboard by a gold pushpin, at eye level from my desk. From Section II, the lines read,

> *Stop this day and night with me, and you shall possess the origin of all poems,*
> *you shall possess the good of the earth and sun (there are millions of suns left)*
> *You shall no longer take things at second or third hand,*
> *nor look through the eyes of the dead, nor feed off specters in books;*
> *You shall not look through my eyes, either, nor take things from me:*
> *You shall listen to all sides, and filter them from ... yourself.*[1]

In the moments recorded in my clinical journals and looking back now, learning to "filter from ... *myself*" turns out to have been one of the most difficult parts of my clinical ethics training. Learning *in* the experience, even when "thrown" by an experience, required careful and rigorous self-reflection – paying attention *to myself* in the experience. The "self" part was the hardest because self-reflection required acknowledging and accepting the idiosyncrasy and situatedness of those experiences as *my* experiences as relevant. I was not prepared for or oriented toward recognizing my experiences as valuable and necessary for understanding on par with other participants' experiences in the unfolding moral moment. I struggled with accepting that one of the fundamental moral elements at stake in my clinical observations was the fact that *I was doing the observations*. I found it difficult, transgressive even, to focus on myself when I was supposed to be learning about Ethics Issues. From the far side of those experiences, it looks like an internalized tendency to remove myself from the scene and scenario – an unwitting participation in a subtle erasure, perhaps rooted in some academically inculcated belief that to make things accessible, applicable, and generalizable requires eliminating specificity, historicity, and particularity. At the time, reflecting on my engagement felt like an illegitimate putting myself forward. Recognizing the value and the validity of my perspectives in making sense of clinical encounters took a lot of unlearning from and with my mentors – from the first days of rounds to the end of the semester encounter with Mrs. Boone described above, and her son's near-catastrophic decompensation which I described in journal entries that follow below.

Acknowledging the moral relevance of my own actions, interactions, understandings, and motivations was a slow process. Even slower was building my practice of doing such self-reflection *in the moments* of clinical involvement rather than alone in my apartment or office hours later. The slowest of all was learning and believing that engaging in practices of rigorous self-reflection is something to do *with others*: that *doing* requires exposing one's unknowing and uncertainty, rather than retreating to claims of expertise. Acknowledging and responding to our own vulnerability becomes part of the necessary communal and professional moral engagement of clinical ethics work.

### *Strangers, Surrenderers, and Self-Reflective Dancers*

The practices of self-reflection and self-education are central to each of the other elements of clinical ethics practice and so they are worth considering carefully. Self-reflection ties deeply to the stranger's practice in approaching a new community or environment – what Schutz describes as the disruption of recognizing the limits of one's own taken-for-granted notions.[2] Self-reflection also mirrors Wolff's surrender-to.[3] Such deliberate and diligent paying attention requires rigorous review of one's assumptions to bracket them and investigate more directly, more immediately what is present. The question I encountered, moving from my MICU experiences and journals to my NICU experiences and journals is how to do that self-reflective work in the midst of my disciplined surrender-to and in my moments of disrupted, befallen surrender in these clinical encounters. Even further, the identification, consideration, and even evaluation of one's values, commitments, beliefs, identity, personality traits, and tendencies *shapes* one's attention, reflections, reasoning, communication, and actions and so creates a moral demand: a need for a reflective responsiveness.

*After a Moment: Recollecting and Reflecting on Meanings and Motivations*

> *The residents both got emergency pages from Avery's room, and for a few weird moments, it felt like a TV medical drama. Everyone took off down the hall, not running, but striding quickly, and I followed along with my heart beating hard and a sick feeling in my stomach. We rounded the corner towards the rooms in the "B-pod" and the first thing to see and hear was Mrs. Boone being held up by three nurses in the main hallway, outside of the pod. She was shaking and wailing, unable to stand as Dr. Carver and the team went through the doors. I didn't know what to do – whether I should stay out in the hall out of the way, whether I should go in, whether I should talk to Mrs. Boone.*

> *I stood by myself by the door for a minute, watching one of the nurses go find a chair for Mrs. Boone, who still couldn't stand. The social worker went to the phone at the reception area in front of B-pod while a nurse came calmly down the hall with a cart full of equipment. I held the door for her into the pod and after another glance at Mrs. Boone's agonized face, I decided to follow the cart and find out what had happened. The hallway in the pod was a little*

*crowded, as was Avery's room. Dr. Carver and the residents were in the room, along with a few nurses and a respiratory therapist. All the other doors in the hall were closed, and I went to stand to one side of the door. I asked what had happened and learned that a mucus plug had gotten stuck in Avery's endotracheal tube. He had turned bright blue in a matter of seconds and wasn't breathing. A nurse (or the RT, I couldn't tell) had suctioned his tube and gotten the plug out, and he was recovering by the time I had joined the team. One of the nurses told another to go tell Mrs. Boone that he was ok, that he was going to be fine, and eventually the wails from outside the pod ceased.*

*Mrs. Boone came down the hall a few minutes later and joined the team in Avery's room. She was still shaking and trying to explain that he had turned so blue so fast. Dr. Carver explained the mucus plug, and that he was better now. Mrs. Boone wanted to know what would happen if he did this again, where the team was going. Carver said they would be back in a little while, and the resident reminded her how quickly they had gotten there. Mrs. Boone seemed a little relieved, remembering that yes, they had gotten there so fast and saying how thankful she was. The team left the pod and went back to rounds, with me in tow: one of the residents made a weak joke about "action and excitement in the NICU," and rounds continued as if nothing had happened.*

*I was so shaken I seriously debated about leaving rounds for the day. I don't imagine seeing babies and families in acute crises such as the Boones had on Wednesday ever gets easy, but I hope that it will perhaps not be so unnerving every time. I found myself amazed once again by the calm of the team and the medical professionals and wondered again at the training and socialization that produces such an organized, choreographed response. Now I find myself wondering whether doing rounds and exposing myself to such events is an intentional part of my socialization and training, and whether it will be less difficult with repetition of similar situations.*

### *Andrea Frolic's Mindful Embodiment*

In looking at the NICU journals, there is a slow shift from reportage to efforts at self-reflection as a deliberate practice. The fits-and-starts, struggles, and discomfort of that process are personal to me in these reflections and yet are not unique to my experiences. Sharing these stories and reflections is personal and interpersonal: as songwriter Joe Henry observes, "The whole process is unfailingly and deeply personal – but the subjects are not."[4] This is Wolff's connection between the historical and the human.[5] I wasn't sure how to accept and make sense of this learning process – the vulnerability of speaking from one's own location, the discomfort with articulating one's self-reflection as a moral element of clinical ethics consultations, despite the encouragement of my teachers to reflect on my own experience.

Even in the moments when I engaged that second order discipline of self-reflection in the writings, when I found myself engaging what was behind and underneath my questions, assumptions, commitments, or actions, I struggled with a kind of shame at what looked like hubris: how could I think that what I did or said might matter? The struggle here was accepting that what I do might matter – and wrestling with a deep, self-protective impulse to say it doesn't – that I'm just a student, an ethics person, myself – all the types of erasure and appeals to a role: it isn't me. What comes out and becomes clear in the conversations with Mrs. Boone is that while my actions and interactions might not matter – they might matter very much. My presence, my response, my words may help or harm in ways I can't discover fully in the moment. As such, if I'm going to be involved, I have to take seriously the fact that my involvement – even as a student, even as an ethics person, even as just me – might matter – which means I have to act *as if* it does. This is a developing practice of being aware of self-reflection and self-education through conversation and interaction with others, so that in clinical encounters, I am aware of my own self enough to be open to the other, to affiliate and attune to them without losing myself.

In the encounter in the NICU and my reflections on it, I was caught by believing that the distinction between the experience and understandings I carried into the clinical encounters and the experiences and understandings others carried meant they were unconnected. I thought that the only ones that mattered for the clinical ethics work – for me as a clinical ethics student – were the experiences and understandings of others. To my dismay and, again, even a kind of shame, though I tried to focus on the patients, families, and clinicians – on conversations with my teachers or what I was reading – I kept coming back to and having to engage with myself and I wasn't sure what to do with those reflections.

The NICU notes expose a kind of self-obscuring that Andrea Frolic described, where the "embodied self quietly slips beneath the surface of the case."[6] Frolic's essay, "Who Are We When We Are Doing What We Are Doing?: The Case for Mindful Embodiment in Ethics Case Consultation" wasn't available when I was student – nor had it been published as I was beginning my work, so I only encountered it later, well into my practice and deeply in this process of revisiting and reflecting on how my clinical ethics practice developed. In reflection on the texts of my NICU Journals, however, Frolic's critique of the hiddenness of the ethics consultant's presence and voice speaks to potential roots of that shame – the de-legitimizing of the consultant's voice in typical ethics literature. Her description of and argument for self-reflective, embodied work thus resonates deeply, offering a frame for reflection on how to be self-reflective.

Frolic's essay explores *situatedness* in clinical ethics consultation, beginning with identifying significant gaps in literature and practice. She looks at embodiment as "more epistemology grounded in body," seeking the interplay of physical, symbolic, intersubjective using critical-interpretive medical anthropology (CIMA) and auto-ethnography (use of one's experiences to integrate and develop theory). Frolic begins with the observation that, "my embodied experiences have been a well-spring of moral insight and of invaluable connection with patients, families, and colleagues I've met during ethics consultation."[7] She continues by more sharply critiquing the gaps in the field:

> it seemed peculiar … that ethics consultants, who are so frequently called to attend to cases that focus on bodies in various states of disability and disease appear to have little intuitive sense of how their own embodied experiences influence their judgments or actions …[8]

Frolic reviews the few avenues within the field of bioethics and clinical ethics that she sees as trying to articulate a more situated, reflective, embodied perspective, but finds each wanting to some degree.

Most notably, Frolic's work critiques Richard Zaner's phenomenology, feminist bioethics, and naturalized bioethics, noting that each continues to position and frame ethics consultants as spectators, as witnesses, or as marginal observers:

> … even as other parties become more fully 'fleshed out' the ethics consultant remains a wraith-like character, a disembodied voice of reason, impervious to personal interests or political pressures, providing unbiased facilitation and principled advice.[9]

Frolic wants to aim research in clinical ethics to "tearing away the veil of neutrality and objectivity" to emphasize and work from the situatedness of the author. Frolic critiques Zaner for being the outsider in his descriptive accounts, though she notes that he had not yet worked out his narrative method in the texts she was engaging. Zaner had worked it out by the time I was a student, and in conversation and engagement with his students and colleagues (including my teachers) and so my exposure and reflections in MICU and NICU were deeply informed by the idea of one's embedded, embodied, particular experiences as morally relevant. And while I also think Zaner was more attuned to and relying on an embodied practice of clinical ethics work than Frolic gives credit for in this account, her critique and even the underlying impetus behind the article are similar: addressing the problematic and typical erasure of the ethics consultant as participant and moral stakeholder in the ethics consultation experience and reporting. The NICU journals illustrate wrestling with that experience – trying to identify and reflect on what is morally or ethically relevant and at stake in the encounter – and where my own or one's own experiences fit in and shape that encounter.

Frolic's "mindful body" approach resonated as a more theoretical and structured representation of some of the practices of paying attention and self-reflection that shaped my clinical ethics education and training. By introducing the practices of CIMA and the three bodies hermeneutic of looking at individual body (lived experience), the social body (metaphors/socially created and understood) and the body politic (body in relation to systems of power and structures)[10], alongside an overview of autoethnography ("method of inquiry and writing that turns one's own experience into the focus of inquiry"[11]), Frolic offered reflective tools for understanding clinical ethics consultation practice *as a clinical ethics consultant*. Rooted in auto-ethnography rather than phenomenology, the parallels in orientation and method ring true as I look back now and consider the challenges of being self-reflective in clinical ethics practice. In fact, the practices which both Frolic and Zaner articulate were among was the hardest lessons I had to learn: I was deeply, unreflectively committed to the ideas of neutrality and critical distance (as demonstrated in parts of the NICU journals and most of the earlier MICU journals). Acknowledging my own moral experience and voicing it in a self-reflective way required *recognizing and unlearning* often un-examined and un-articulated commitments and practices. I *struggled* to do that work, despite constant encouragement from Mark and Stuart to consider the *why* and *how* behind the *what* of my attention. Even as self-reflection itself became a focus of attention, these student journals reflect more of the disembodied observer, more of the removed or distanced reflections, or the intellectualized questions that emerged in trying to account for both my observations and my experiences of observing.

Frolic's work helped articulate why the emerging self-reflection of the NICU journals matters: given how few examples of self-reflective writing there have been and given that "scholarly" and "objective" writing and analysis is so prevalent, self-effacement has to be *unlearned*, actively resisted as one is *thrown* by experiences, trembling. The concern for speaking of one's own experiences emerges in these NICU journals as a painful vulnerability of clinical ethics work, facing the question of "What if I'm wrong? What if it's just me?" Yet, like the possibility of the catch that may emerge from the befallen-ness of being thrown into surrender, profound vulnerability carries the profound possibility for openness and learning. The willingness to speak of those experiences – even if it might be just me, even if I might be wrong – becomes part of the responsibility in clinical ethics. I can only learn whether my experience is interpreted as shared or idiosyncratic, reliable or suspect, relevant to others or only to myself (which is not to say irrelevant) *by speaking*, by engaging as what Frolic identifies as an embodied participant, from what Wolff would call the "ineluctable boundaries of his (sic) historicity," unique location and space.[12]

The traces of recognition, the growing acceptance of my own embodied and particular experience as a legitimate and even necessary position from which to engage and reflect on clinical ethics practice, unfolded slowly during my NICU rounds – a type of unintended auto-ethnography. The practice of subjecting my own experiences to verbatim presentation and reflection with others became more deliberately immediate in the NICU rounds as I tried to be explicit to myself about what I was observing, thinking, and doing *while* doing it – as well as in the conversations and journals after.

*Too Serious for Trial and Error*

*Talking with Bliton about reflective/intentional behavior while trying to identify what matters; what counts as facts, and what counts as evidence in making decision; what is important to those involved, about how to be reflective in these interactions, and I was thinking afterwards of one of the last babies we visited on rounds, baby Avery. Mom and grandparents were in the room. After Dr. Carver talked about moving towards bottle-feeding, Granddad made a joke about "Put a little Bud Light in the bottle and he'll be set." I was standing next to him and joked back saying, "Not that kind of bottle." He chuckled and we smiled and then I froze inside – wondering whether it was appropriate for me to be talking to and joking with this man. He made a general joke (albeit, a weak one) and I, by responding to it and joking back, may have been intruding myself upon him. Maybe I crossed some boundary of appropriate interaction. Or maybe I was instinctively responding to his discomfort with the situation, and so behaving appropriately. The latter sounds better, and I think is somewhat accurate, but I still don't know for sure. I did get a sense of discomfort from the man – which was reinforced later. Mom and Grandma were talking about how different the skin around the feeding tube looked. Grandma said something about wanting to see it, or looking forward to seeing it, and Granddad leaned towards me and said, in a stage whisper, "I think I can wait to see it," and then chuckled. Why would I say this indicated discomfort? Well, humor is often one way of dealing with the difficult or the upsetting. It's the whistling in the dark or laughing at fear ... there is so little that is funny about a NICU baby that when Granddad attempted a lame joke, I knew, without even really thinking about it, that he was trying to cope with the situation by making the joke. Because I joked back with him, he made his second joke directly to me.*

*What would I say I had picked up in all of this? That while Mom and Grandma seemed comfortable with the details, with talking to the doctors, with the physicality of the baby's complications, the Granddad seemed uncomfortable with all of it. What would I do with this information? Is this an insight into how to talk with this family? Could I perhaps have used this to direct discussions with the different adults in the family – i.e., speaking in more general and less descriptive terms with the Granddad, while being as explicit and direct as possible with Mom and Grandma, since they appeared to comfortable with and perhaps take comfort in that kind of communication.*

*So, that still doesn't answer whether or not it was appropriate for me to interact with the Granddad like that since I am not a part of the care team. However, I would say that my response was appropriate from one person to another – though I think this is perhaps the kind of thing that requires that ongoing, simultaneous reflection Dr. Bliton was talking about. In this case, no one else was responding to his uncomfortable humor. Perhaps they would have if I hadn't, but perhaps not, and how awful that would have been – the already uncomfortable man made more uncomfortable by the lack of reaction to his joke. So anyway, good or bad, I'm glad I did respond.*

*It still, however, raises that issue of reflection in my activities and words. I reacted and responded without thinking about it and have been wondering about and thinking about it ever since. If I had been invited in to talk to the family, that joke might have been an opening to ask the Granddad about how he felt hearing the detailed, explicit description of his grandchild's condition, and maybe how he felt about or what he thought about the child's condition, treatment, future possibilities, etc. It might have been an opening, as well, to include the Mom and Grandma in that discussion. Which makes me wonder how one initiates such conversations – with individual family members alone or in a group setting with all of them? I imagine it depends largely on the family dynamics, but it is my understanding that having all the people involved communicate is important or a goal.*

*The question I have is how to become aware of the family dynamics. Do you fly by the seat of your pants at the beginning, while maintaining self-reflection, and adapt or change direction according to the circumstances? Again, that seems logical, but leads to the question of how one develops the practical wisdom to do that a) effectively and b) benignly. This seems like too serious of a situation to allow trial-and-error to be the method of choice. The effects of error seem too potentially detrimental. Yet, it seems like there will be errors in judgment on how to initiate or proceed with conversations. So, how does one learn how to approach family members (or doctors, or nurses) about tricky topics like this?*

Frolic argues for seeing auto-ethnography as an *ethical practice* "promoting greater transparency in the production of knowledge and a more robust exploration of the agency of the researcher/author (including the influences of lived experiences and social and political contexts on the choices made in the context of research)."[13] She gives a beautiful metaphor of learning to dance and the importance of the experiences that shape our commitments, contexts, and choices. Frolic writes, from her perspective as a dancer,

One can read about dance, one can watch dance, but one does not become a dancer in any way other than dancing. Similarly, one can learn the theories of ethics and analyze cases, but one can only become an ethics consultant by practicing ethics consultation, preferably under the tutelage of a skilled practitioner who can transmit both the analytic and embodied tradition of the practice.[14]

Frolic's dance example captures my experience in the NICU particularly regarding the invitation to participate in the case conference regarding Avery Boone.

### The Occasion for Practice Emerged

*A little nervous. Ok, very nervous. This morning before rounds I was talking with Dr. Carver about how the weekend had gone, and he said it had been fairly quiet, that they had no admissions on Sunday, but that some of the babies were fairly sick. He mentioned that Avery Boone had gram negative sepsis and had a difficult weekend, that he looked like he could die yesterday. He said that they were having a care conference this afternoon, and that I was welcome to join them if I wanted to. He said that Avery's mom had asked him whether these treatments were heroic and should maybe be stopped, and he told her that they were not heroic, that most babies with his condition needed this kind of care, and that some needed more. Dr. Carver said the father was in town which was why they had scheduled the care conference for today. There was some discussion during rounds about postponing it until Dr. Liu could participate, but after discussion, the mother and father decided to have it today before the father left town.*

*So, I struggled all during rounds and in the early afternoon about attending this conference. On the one hand, I was nervous about doing so without direct permission from Dr. Bliton or Dr. Finder – both of whom are out of the country. I didn't know if they would think it appropriate for me to be there with the family, even as an observer. On the other hand, this is an opportunity for me to see what happens in a care conference, what kinds of things are discussed, who participates, how the conversations move, and what kinds of things matter to the people at the conference. I also did not want to appear ungrateful for the opportunity or unwilling to learn more, so I accepted the invitation to attend the conference. I am getting ready to head that way in a few moments, and will do some more writing and thinking about it when I get back. I don't really know what to expect, even though this is a child and family I have followed since the beginnings of my rounds.*

I had been studying, engaging, reflecting under tutelage and guidance and yet it wasn't until the occasion for practice emerged and I responded on my own that I felt the fresh weight of responsibility for how my self-reflections shaped my actions. When the occasion for practice emerged, I felt unready to "begin," as if I needed more preparation, though I realized and accepted, that I had already begun, that I had been preparing through paying attention and self-reflection all along. I recognized that in the moment of clinical ethics *practice* (i.e., *my participation* in the care conference for Avery and after), *my involvement* required agile self-reflection and mindfulness, embodied awareness in the encounter, necessary for writing of and sharing of reflections after the fact.

The NICU and Avery's care conference thus stand as a pivotal set of experiences – both the recognition of embodied self as locus/starting point of reflection – taking seriously the practices of paying attention *and* the recognition that sharing stories of one's experiences with others is one way that the practice of the self-reflection works to avoid being caught in and reinforcing its own commitments. Frolic argues that

> mindful embodiment facilitates greater transparency and accountability in the work as consultants learn to articulate precisely who they are, what they do, and why they do what they do. An embodied epistemology enables consultants to model self-reflection and appropriate disclosure of personal concerns, feelings, and values in the consultation process, empowering stakeholders to be open and honest too.[15]

The added insights from Frolic's emphasis on intuitions and emotions and comportment as sources/locus of moral epistemology helps explain the need to subject individual experiences to rigorous self-reflection and dialogue with others. Although embodied self-reflection in the moments of a dance, of a consultation, is necessary, this sort of self-reflection and dialogue requires that we test those reflections, in communications with others – exploring the *interpersonal* through the access point of the personal. In this way, to be responsible in self-reflection also requires being open to probing and questions from others – not as a test for some objective truth/realness of one's embodied experience but for the meaning of one's experiences, which then leads to understanding what might be going on in current circumstances and contexts.

To escape the potential solipsism of mindful inquiry into individual body/lived experience, Frolic insists that self-reflection is something to be exercised and done with others, placing her firmly within – and richly expanding – a multi-disciplinary tradition with Schutz, Wolff, Zaner, and others. While this tradition recognizes that the disruption of encounters and engagement with others often prompt self-reflection, it also insists that reflecting with others can improve the *practice and discipline and rigor* of self-reflection by creating and even requiring the kind of disruption that one may habitually avoid on one's own. This points to the connection between self-refection and self-education as parts of clinical ethics practice.

*I Could Write a Book ...*

*I spoke last week with Dr. Bliton about the difficulties in writing about experiences in rounds. That was spurred in part by the challenges in writing about the care conference and in part by discussions from Seminar. The question keeps circling in my head about 'how do I write about an event in a way that does justice to that event and to those involved?' The care conference, for example, was an hour and a half of conversation, involving mostly Dr. Carver, Mr. and Mrs. Boone, and Dr. Leon. It took me three days and almost nine single-spaced pages to write about the bare-bones of what happened – to construct a report of the event. I have only touched the edges of the most obvious things that happened, or were said. Each of those mini-events within the care conference holds a wealth of details, nuances, and profound issues that I feel ought to be addressed, yet I'm not sure if I can fully address them.*

*I feel like I could write a book on nothing but the different words, different uses of language that shaped the atmosphere of the conference. I could probably write another book on the myriad of conflicting emotions my involvement with this family has produced – culminating in but extending beyond the moments of the care conference. So how do I learn from these encounters? Where do I begin, or perhaps before that, where do I want to go? Or perhaps, which of those questions deserves priority in deciding how I write about this experience and others like it?*

*I ask this last question because it strikes me as important to figure out how to approach writing about clinical experiences. I have usually begun by picking one aspect, one event and following where it leads. For example, describing a conversation about a surgery patient in the NICU leads to thinking about conversations about surgical residents which leads to thinking and writing about the conflicts between the two groups of residents who are caring for the same patient. The writing sort of spirals outwards, and sometimes back in again or sometimes spirals off into another direction. The direction of most of my writing seems more organic than disciplined or planned.*

*Is that the best way to approach thinking and writing about these kinds of experiences – following the spiraling constellations of interconnected thought? Or ought I be looking for specific features in these events, something to direct the way I think and write about them? Is there some unifying theme or structure in what I'm observing, experiencing, and trying to relate? If so, I haven't found it yet, but that doesn't mean it's not there. It seems to me so far that each of these events has its own logic and structure, yet they are all related, some differently than others. It's like the six-degrees of separation game – how is X related to Y and why? And how do I explain that relationship?*

*I guess my frustration is that sitting now, at the end of this semester's rounds, I am looking for some sense of closure, of completion, even as I have the sneaking suspicion there is no closure, no completion. How does that fit in my education and training? I still have questions*

*about what happens in the NICU and why. I still wonder every few days how Avery Boone is,
I'm still trying to make sense of what I am learning and how I am learning it. And I am still
trying to grow accustomed to the need for self-reflection, to focus intently on myself and what
I am doing. It's a lot easier to pay attention to what others are doing. It's more complicated to
examine my goals, my experiences, my relations to others in this project, and what I can and
should think about and do with these experiences. This is part of what makes the writing difficult. How many of my personal idiosyncrasies shape what I think and write, and since they
do shape how I approach my experiences, can I or should I bracket them? Are they useful
lenses or something to be overcome or pushed aside? As I am trying to think about my larger
paper for this semester's internship, I am trying to figure out not only what to write about,
but how to write about it. I'm pretty sure there can be more than one correct answer to these
questions. I'm just trying to think about what might be appropriate or fitting answers – if
there is some kind of starting point that is better than others.*

*I've decided the hardest papers, essays, reflections, whatever, to write are those in which I
am most invested. On a topic or a question about which I care deeply, I am almost frozen
when I try to write, and never satisfied with the final result. I can understand the stasis over
the final result. In one sense, the most basic I suppose, there is a concern over how it will be
received, after I have invested so much time, energy, thought into it. Behind that, however, is
the fear that inhibits the initial writing – that I don't know enough to write it, or that I don't
have enough of a grasp on the subject, or that I'm missing something important, something
obvious.*

### Reflecting on NICU Journals and the Practice of Self-Education

Years after writing those reflections, more than ten years after discovering Frolic's essay about
the value of ethics consultants' experiences, I still wonder about and worry about the value of
self-reflection and the validity of working from my own perspectives into the broader field. How
can I learn from my unique, *sui generis* experiences in ways that resonate with or have relevance
to others' experiences? How can I learn from what and how I know without making it all about
me and what and how *I* know? Especially in a field and tradition that is still deeply committed to
procedural forms of knowing,[16] which does not tolerate the subtle variations of the individual or
personal – except in passing. "Oh, of course this is about unique people, individual lives, but how
are we going to operationalize this across a system? Or assure the same quality outcomes so we
can measure our efficacy?" Facing an increasing juggernaut of professionalism that pushes toward
the universal, the standardizable, the replicable and reliable, offering and owning one's particular
perspective as one's own still feels rebellious, risky, and vulnerable.

And yet, practice of articulating and accounting for one's perspective in the clinical encounter
is also part of the work of clinical ethics consultants modeling this practice for those *in* the consultations, as Frolic points out. Stakeholders – whether patients, families, or clinicians – are often
similarly uncertain about the relevance and value of past experiences and understandings to present moment. They, too, are desperate to be heard and worried they won't be – wondering if their
perspective will be recognized as important, especially if it doesn't fit in more dominant modes of
communication, expressions, or worldviews in healthcare.

So, I reflect on and resist the voices of internalized and external critics who dismiss the embodied and individuated as idiosyncratic and irrelevant. It is no pleasant business; and it feels like
having to excavate oneself from sedimented weight of traditions and communities that never quite
fit, searching for fellow travelers and voices that resonate, from any direction.

Fortunately, such voices do exist, and in the wild serendipity of the universe,[17] they might be discovered in the moment they are needed. In that completely accidental way, while reflecting on the challenges presented by this project and revisiting Frolic's invitation to embodied self-reflection, I came across an article containing just such a voice from just such a fellow traveler, considering the idea of self-education.

### Harald Ofstad and Self-Education in Moral Development

I encountered Harald Ofstad, a Norwegian philosopher, through a reading assigned for our Cedars-Sinai iteration of the Seminar in Clinical Philosophy: "Education vs Growth in Moral Development."[18] Published in *the Monist* in 1974, Ofstad articulates the value of self-reflection and stresses the necessary influence of self-education and individual experience in moral development. This approach harmonized beautifully with the questions of how to fulfill Frolic's – and my teachers' – calls for self-reflection as a communal activity. Since moral development turns out to be a key theme for education and training in clinical ethics practice, it was surprisingly helpful as I reflect on my own education and training. Written more than 30 years *before* I started my clinical observations and encountered almost 20 years *after* I began by "finding my way up the hill" to the Center for Clinical and Research Ethics at Vanderbilt University, Ofstad's work articulates, in a different language, key themes about the responsibility for and work of clinical ethics consultation present in Schutz, Wolff, and Zaner, along with Frolic and my own growing moral and clinical sensibilities.

Ofstad's work in this article explores the idea of moral education as helping people become "autonomous and responsible moral agents who take serious things seriously."[19] He argues that the elements of such development occur through social growth and interaction more than from didactic methods or the indoctrination of information (though each mode of teaching requires attention and can serve in particular contexts). Even though education may help stimulate or support such growth, Ofstad argues that

> self-education, i.e., rational and sensitive examination of important happenings and the way in which we react to them can further, in a more or less indirect way, the fulfillment of the goal (of having people become morally responsible agents) especially during maturity.[20]

For Ofstad, the value is learning through autonomous inquiry: the goal of moral education is not memorization and application of moral rights and wrongs, but rather to allow the agent to learn and discover. He continues, explaining that

> our moral beliefs are more or less uncertain. For our moral insight is fallible and our beliefs may be based on failure or incomplete knowledge. Granting this, we ought to conclude that it is both morally and intellectually irresponsible to moral education as a communication of what we pretend to know of moral truths. Moral beliefs should be taught by way of rational discussion between the teacher and his (sic) pupils.[21]

Ofstad argues that the process of "trying to find out which norms and values one ought to accept and how one ought to apply them is valuable" because it is central to the development of one's identity as a person: like Frolic's dancer or the ethics consultant – figuring out how we do what we do by doing it, and figuring out who we are when we're doing it. For Ofstad,

> the goal of moral education is not only to make people act rightly, since that doesn't take into account the value of autonomous moral inquiry. Neither ought the goal be to only make

people into maximally independent decision-makers, since that goal doesn't take into account the value of acting rightly. The goal must be to stimulate the development of autonomous, rational, and sensitive decision-makers who deliberate within a frame of certain fundamental norms and values forming the minimum conditions of any acceptable moral system.[22]

We're not looking for machines to calculate algorithms of correct behavior – we're looking for morally engaged people.

Part of what resonates is Ofstad's account of the characteristics of an autonomous and responsible decision-making, "our ideal moral agent," because the elements he lays out for a responsible moral agent are applicable to one's activities and development as a clinical ethics consultant. For example, Ofstad says the "agent should have critically examined the moral norms and values which he tends to accept and should be disposed to continuous examination of the kind,"[23] which has parallels to the stranger's examination of recipes and the CIMA work that Frolic describes in her reflections on the situatedness of the ethics consultant. Ofstad explains that the agent's critical examination should also include the "empirical presuppositions of those norms and values and should be disposed to pay serious attention to the facts which, according to his norm and values system, are relevant to the problems with which he is confronted."[24] Echoing Wolff's concern for attention to the problem at hand and learning what is relevant during the surrender-to and even the surrender-and-catch, Ofstad's work further parallels Wolff in the insistence that the agent "should be open to arguments and willing to modify his judgments and to examine the relevant facts, norms, and values in an impartial, cautious, and critical manner."[25] The willingness to suspend or release the things we *know* reflexively is part of the moral development Ofstad argues is available to – and necessary for everyone.

The meaning that resonates here is understanding this emphasis on rational, self-critical impartial is not an abstracted "view from nowhere" of the kind Frolic warns against, rather the meaning is what grows in recognizing that we all come *from somewhere* and have a responsibility to be as aware of, engaged with, and critically reflective about our norms and values as we can. And Ofstad is clear that he thinks we can and should engage that responsibility. This is a challenge, as I wrote in my first week of NICU rounds:

*So, What Can I Figure Out from These?*

*Figuring out how people know what they say they know – how do you do this? Rather, how do I do this? How do I know what Dr. Carver says is accurate, or what the resident presents is accurate? And useful – i.e., in deciding what to do about the care of this child?*

*I have to assume the doctor knows what he is talking about because he is a trained NICU doctor, he is an attending, which (in theory) means he knows enough to teach, and he has the experience of doing this for a long time.*

*Can I make any guesses about his assumptions/leanings/mindset based on what I see? Well, what do I see? What can I figure out from these?*

Ofstad notes the situational and ambiguous lenses through which we necessarily understand the facts, norms, and values and that "we cannot exclude the possibility that some of our personality traits, as well as traits of the society to which we belong, may influence our selection of and interpretation of them."[26] He argues (like Frolic) that the more careful and attentive we are to those traits, and how they shape our decisions and activities, the more we may "be able to check their distracting influence."[27] As such, Ofstad offers two more claims that are relevant to the development of and practice of clinical ethics consultants. First that the ideal moral agent should "have a realistic picture of himself, his feelings, desires, attributes, prejudices, reaction-tendencies and of the way in which these may influence his selection, interpretation, and balancing of facts, norms, and values."[28] Second, that the agent "should also be disposed to actually confront himself – in the course of his decision-making with such data concerning the way these personality traits may influence his decision-making."[29] Ofstad's observation mapped directly onto some of the work my teachers did with me in those early weeks of the NICU observations.

*Isn't That What Normally Happens?*

*One woman, Avery's mother, whose parents were in the room with her last week, and with whom I interacted, is one example. As I noticed last week, she seemed deeply interested and involved in the details about and care of her son. This week that was made even more apparent. She was in the room when the house-staff came by on Monday, and asked them questions, talking about how she had just changed the bandage on her son's giant omphalocele, the sac containing his internals organs protruding through his abdomen. She and the nurse (the nurse especially) badgered the house-staff and Dr. Desai into being very clear about what the next steps were in the infant's care and insisted that they all look at the new skin growth. The mother showed no awkwardness about her son's condition, or sadness, and was neither subservient or indifferent to what Dr. Desai and the residents had to say. She seemed engaged and excited about the futures they were talking about, and she seemed grateful for the care she and her son had received from the team. Before we left the room, she presented one of the interns with a box of cookies and a note addressed to them, the "Red Team."*

*When Dr. Bliton and I were talking after rounds, she came up in conversation, and he described her as brave. I remember thinking that the term was both odd and apt. Odd because why is it especially brave for a mother to be taking care of her son? Isn't that what normally happens? In my corner of the universe, where in my family and my family of friends, babies are considered a blessing and parenthood is an assumed goal, yes it is. But in that corner of the universe, most people who become parents are married, well-settled, with a big support network, and almost all of the babies I have known have been healthy, hearty, and happy. Even knowing on an intellectual level that this is not the case with many people, my background led me to assume that people will naturally take responsibility for loving and caring for their child, no matter what the circumstances. One week in the NICU is enough to show how narrow that vision is, and I think it began shifting before that first day of rounds was over. Instead of wondering – abstractly – how a parent could not take care of their child no matter how sick or premature, I found myself wondering how they pull themselves together to do it. How could these parents not just give up, shut down, shut themselves away from any love or responsibility for a child with such difficulties?*

In my NICU rounds, I found myself confronting any number of beliefs and values that I didn't even know I carried because they were so taken-for-granted from previous experiences (or a lack of experiences), that I only recognized them in or after the moment was concerning, disconcerting even. I realized how much the values and commitments I held had influenced the meanings I assigned to others actions and words, how much my "recipes" for being in the world, and my "provinces of meaning" shaped my understandings in this strange new land of the NICU.[30] It kept happening too: the recurrent discovery that what I thought I knew and believed were both important *and* were shaping how I made sense of the new experiences. Thus, self-reflection and ongoing learning turned out to be neither a finite process nor a solitary activity.

### *Always More or Less Dissatisfied: Ofstad's 10th Characteristic of the Moral Agent*

As important as I recognize that Ofstad's articulation of growing – and confronting – a realistic self-understanding to be, he described another characteristic of the moral agent that resonated most strongly with clinical ethics training – such that I laughed out loud with delighted fellow-feeling the first time I read it. Ofstad begins by noting that the moral agent

> should be open to different arguments and willing to modify his judgments. This condition of maturity is part of a more comprehensive attitude of inquiry subjecting one's total worldview, including one's norms and values system and its applications, to continual re-examination.[31]

Ofstad then lays out his 10th characteristic of the ideal moral agent: that "the agent continually subjects his moral development to critical examination, tries to deepen and broaden his perspective, and *is always more or less dissatisfied with himself and his relations with the world.*"[32]

The relief-of-recognition is what prompted the hilarity. Ofstad's 10th characteristic – in a nutshell – is the parallel to the orientation of the stranger, or the disrupted but focused attention of the surrender-to: being aware of and recognizing one's own particular moral norms and values, and the personality traits and attributes that influence them, and subjecting them to constant re-examination. What Schutz describes as disruption from engagement with the strangeness of the approached group (and recognition of oneself as a stranger in this context), Ofstad puts forth as a matter-of-fact, necessary practice. And, growth in moral understanding is the "catch," brought on by what Wolff describes as the crisis, the overwhelm of the surrender. All three, however, illustrate a common theme that emerged across the student experiences of Seminar, MICU, and NICU rounds: paying attention to the received notions/recipes/taken-for-granted values and norms is a potentially overwhelming discipline but necessary for responsible engagement, understanding, right action within the world – and it is a never-ending process. The choice to enact that responsibility – to engage with one's own values and motivations in order to explore and discover with others – is a recurrent one: encounters with others, especially in clinical ethics work, bring the constant invitation to inquiry rather than reliance on convention and the taken-for-granted. Whether or not the ethics consultant responds is a matter of personal responsibility, ever in question.

### *Will I Miss Understanding If I Don't Ask?*

> *I have decided that doing rounds is sometimes like walking into a conversation that has been going on for a long time. You don't know who started it – what the initial reason for the conversation was – and you are not sure who said what before you enter the room. If you listen carefully and watch people closely, you think you might be able to pick up on what's going on. Yet, you are uncertain about whether the things you pick up on are important. Are they the main points of the conversation – speaking to the core of the matter? Or are they sidebars? Personal flourishing for attention? Tiny details that shift focus from the main issue or tiny details that inform the main issue?*

> *You try to figure out how other people think the conversation is going. This person is frowning. Is she upset, or is she concentrating? This person looks tired. Is he tired from*

*lack of sleep, or tired of the conversation? This person looks uncomfortable. Is she un-comfortable because she heard something unpleasant? Because she doesn't like the con-versation? Is she uncomfortable at all? Then the self-evaluating questions emerge: what if this woman is not uncomfortable at all, but I am, and I am projecting my own discomfort onto her? What if I missed the things that are important, or in my ignorance, miss under-standing the entire core of the conversation? How can I find out what is going on in the conversation in a reliable or sound way? Am I intruding if I ask for a recap? Will I miss understanding if I don't ask?*

The relief I had in reading Ofstad was recognizing his explanation that self-reflection and self-education *require* a rigorous dialectical stance: both bracing for impact of disruption and being willing to be dislodged from one's foundation/safe-haven. Thus, moral agency requires intellectual openness and a kind of steadfastness that distinguishes between instruction and education. The former he describes as the imparting of information or skills. He is most concerned with the latter: "rational dialogue" with emphasis on self-analysis and reflection, performed "not as an intellectual game, but so that he feels the conclusions in his bones."[33] Ofstad looks for the student who recog-nizes these endeavors, the *practice* as something that matters, something serious.

Ofstad considers maturity as a stage of moral development marked by realizing one's identity and interactions with others as active and serious concerns. He argues for self-education as the primary mode of learning here, in which

> one subjects one's ethical systems, the degree of rationality and of identification with others that one has achieved as well as one's ability to transform one's moral intentions in actions, to critical examination from time to time, repairing ones daily mind at the search station of one's better mind, as it were.[34]

Being open and willing to engage through intentional, diligent examination or reflection on the relevance and fitting-ness of one's taken-for-granted recipes requires having the moral maturity to do so. Ofstad writes, "for it is partly by trying out different activities that the individual finds out what he wants and is able to do, thereby gradually developing self-respect and identity."[35] Moral development and one's integration and identity as a moral agent (in our context, as an ethics con-sultant) grows through both social and individual experiences, honest critique and accepting the risk that finding them insufficient or inadequate might require different learning or action.

### Shared Self-Reflection and Communal Self-Education in Clinical Ethics Practice

Reading Frolic and Ofstad, I find frames for understanding the connections and meanings woven between the individuated experiences of my clinical training and the requirement for ongoing en-gagement within community. The idea was then – and is now, still – that reflection is a practice one engages in *with others* – inviting them to probe, push, and question, along with us, what is taken-for-granted, assumed, essential, superfluous, historical/individual, or human/shared.

Thus, as Frolic suggests, self-reflection is both a necessary precursor to and a part of the on-going practice of clinical ethics, and part of how we prepare for, perform, and demonstrate this practice to others – including to those with whom we are consulting. The clinical ethics consultant can demonstrate her practice of self-reflection as an intentional model that invites others to reflect on themselves and their experiences in conversation and in the consultation. The challenge for the ethics consultant (or clinician or patient) is being self-reflective enough to recognize the limitations of her received notions – even the ones that authorize her presence in the consultation.

Similarly, Ofstad seeks a kind of rigor and discipline in self-education with others, which makes possible a shared, universal human connection or experience through which understanding emerges, though doing so requires acknowledging others' locations, others' assumptions, may shake up the stability of one's own foundations. Ofstad suggests, optimistically but perhaps not unrealistically, that as moral agents, humans can and ought to develop this practice of self-reflection and the discipline of self-education – acknowledging one's historical location and specific taken-for-granted assumptions even if it means never being quite at ease again.

The challenge and question, illustrated by the increasingly reflexive self-reflections in my NICU journals, becomes how to be self-reflective in the moments of clinical encounters. What does it feel like or look like to practice of self-reflection and self-education with others? How can I bracket and hold assumptions and received notions in reserve to consider fully what is present here and now? How do I, as the clinical ethics consultant, become attuned to the question, the concern, the idea, the other people in front of me? These questions of self-reflection become – in practice – questions around affiliation and attunement in moral encounters with others.

## Notes

1  Whitman, Walt (1855). Song of Myself. In *Leaves of Grass (Deathbed Edition)*. New York, NY: Random House Modern Library: 1993. § 2.
2  Schutz, Alfred (1944). The stranger: An essay in social psychology. *American Journal of Sociology* 49(6):499–507.
3  Wolff, Kurt H. (1976). Surrender and catch: Experience and inquiry today. In *Boston Studies in the Philosophy and History of Science*, vol. 51. Dordrecht: Springer.
4  Henry, Joe (2019). Personal notes from live performance/interview. *The Drop* at the Grammy Museum, Los Angeles, CA. December 12, 2019.
5  Wolff, 24.
6  Frolic. Andrea (2011). Who are we when we are doing what we are doing? The case for mindful embodiment in ethics case consultation. *Bioethics* 25 (7):370–382. 374 fn 24
7  *Ibid.* 372.
8  *Ibid.*
9  *Ibid.* 374.
10  *Ibid.* 374–375.
11  *Ibid.* 376.
12  Wolff, 24.
13  *Ibid.* 376.
14  *Ibid.* 379–380.
15  *Ibid.* 380.
16  Friedrich, Annie B. (2018). The pitfalls of proceduralism: An exploration of the goods internal to the practice of clinical ethics consultation. *HEC Forum* 30 (4):389–403.
17  Henry, Joe and Currin, Grayson Haver. Joe Henry's Next Second Chance. *National Public Radio* interview. November 15, 2019. https://www.npr.org/2019/11/15/779415463/joe-henry-album-gospel-according-to-water-cancer-second-chance
18  Ofstad, Harald (1974). Education versus growth in moral development. *The Monist* 58 (4):581–599.
19  *Ibid.* 581.
20  *Ibid.*
21  *Ibid.* 582.
22  *Ibid.* 584.
23  *Ibid.* 585.
24  *Ibid.*
25  *Ibid.* 585.
26  *Ibid.* 586.
27  *Ibid.*
28  *Ibid.*
29  *Ibid.*

30 Schutz, Alfred (1962). Choosing among Projects of Action. In Maurice Natanson (ed.), *Collected Papers of Alfred Schutz: The Problem of Social Reality*, vol. 1. The Hague: Martinus Nijhoff. pp. 67–98.
31 *Ibid.* 588.
32 Ofstad, 588.
33 *Ibid.* 589.
34 *Ibid.* 596–597.
35 *Ibid.* 597.

## Bibliography

Friedrich, Annie B. (2018). The pitfalls of proceduralism: An exploration of the goods internal to the practice of clinical ethics consultation. *HEC Forum* 30 (4):389–403.

Frolic, Andrea (2011). Who are we when we are doing what we are doing? The case for mindful embodiment in ethics case consultation. *Bioethics* 25 (7):370–382.

Henry, Joe and Currin, Grayson Haver (2019). Joe Henry's next second chance. *National Public Radio Interview*. November 15, 2019. https://www.npr.org/2019/11/15/779415463/joe-henry-album-gospel-according-to-water-cancer-second-chance

Henry, Joe (2019). Personal notes from live performance/interview. *The Drop* at the Grammy Museum, Los Angeles, CA. December 12, 2019.

Ofstad, Harald (1974). Education versus growth in moral development. *The Monist* 58 (4):581–599.

Schutz, Alfred (1944). The stranger: An essay in social psychology. *American Journal of Sociology* 49 (6):499–507.

Schutz, Alfred (1962). Choosing Among Projects of Action. In Maurice Natanson (ed.), *Collected Papers of Alfred Schutz: The Problem of Social Reality*, vol 1. The Hague: Martinus Nijhoff. pp. 67–98.

Whitman, Walt. (1855). Song of Myself. In *Leaves of Grass (Deathbed Edition)*. New York, NY: Random House Modern Library: 1993.

Wolff, Kurt H. (1976). Surrender and Catch: Experience and Inquiry Today. In *Boston Studies in the Philosophy and History of Science*, vol. 51. Dordrecht: Springer.

# 4 Affiliation and Attunement and Extra-Ordinary Discourse

## Pivotal and Grounding Orientations: Attunement, Understanding, and What Is Meant by "Ethics"

Attunement seems like a funny word in the context of clinical ethics. I started off thinking it had a kind of hippie, New-Age feel to it, as if somehow slightly disconnected from the seriousness and rigor required by the issues and concerns that arise in clinical encounters. Yet, over time, and especially during my clinical ethics training with the MOMS trial,[1] I learned that attunement is a key to the orientation and practical activities that compose a *method* of clinical ethics consultation. I started to understand attunement as a practice with multiple, distinguishable – if not always separable – activities and communications with other people.

First, attunement requires carefully informed attention to the actual unfolding circumstances within which crucial, and at times disruptive, conversations and questions occur. That attention emerges from an invitation into the situation at hand.[2] Being invited creates a second requirement: the careful and respectful attention to *the other persons* for whom those questions matter, with whom I am in conversation. A third is reflective attention to how I'm paying attention to and developing my understanding of these others, with them in their own circumstances. This evokes an invitation to myself – and a moral demand to be open and responsive.[3] In these activities, attunement becomes a practice of embodied moral inquiry that is performative, iterative, self-aware, and reflexive, embodied in and reflected on throughout those activities.

These three key activities – attending to circumstances, attending to others, and attending to self – are dynamic and susceptible to shifts in relation to the circumstances and likewise in their relevance to each other. However, the practice of each can be articulated and be deployed intentionally, included in a method for learning about and understanding what is at stake in a particular moment, in a particular encounter, for the particular other(s) involved.

These elements of attunement in clinical ethics consultation are not flying blind, trial-and-error as I feared in my early experiences of training. Rather, each element unfolds in deeply social and moral encounters and thus require preparation regarding the specific contexts of engagement. In my ethics interviews and surgery observations in the MOMS trial it became clear that attunement, as a method, *can* be prepared for and anticipated, imagined, and revised and reimagined.[4]

Take, for example, the outlines and questions of my "mental notes for prenatal surgery consults." These were developed over time as I observed and participated in more MOMS interviews. They were my preparation and structure, my education and organization for the times I would be responsible for the conversations and engagement with the issues and concerns that came up. They contributed components necessary to the "actual" work of engagement. Even so, each engagement was different and elicited different practices of preparation and listening. I carried those notes with

DOI: 10.4324/9781003354864-8

me in a folder to the interviews I led by myself, although I did so as a talisman in hand, rather than a checklist to complete. The questions reminded me what had mattered to others in this context, what I might need to pay attention to in this particular moment, with these particular people. My "mental notes" were the preparation and structure that allowed me to be open and attentive to whatever questions, concerns, issues, hopes, fears, needs or expectations each couple brought to the conversation. The questions were not a safety net – more like a tether in recognition that sometimes such engagements could become disruptive in unanticipated ways, a divining rod to get me back to some of the underlying concerns. Yet even with preparation of previous research and insights from others who have experienced their own versions of the circumstances at hand, methods of attunement are *discovered* in the encounter and *responsive* to what emerges in the encounter with those other people.[5]

### *Texts on Attunement*

Reflecting on my experiences from beginning to conduct ethics consultations on my own brings into sharper focus questions about what attunement *looks like* and how I could recognize and develop those skills in my practice. The story of "Me and the Moms" that follows is about my observations and participation in interviews and surgeries as these took place during the MOMS trial. This kind of story represents the best way I have found to illustrate those varieties of clinical attunement and the challenges encountered in those activities of becoming attuned, both to the circumstances and the others with whom one is engaged. In reviewing and reflecting on these experiences I reconnected with some of the primary texts that helped make sense out of the idea of attunement.

For questions of method, both Richard Zaner's essay, "Phenomenology and the Clinical Event,"[6] and Pierre Bourdieu's essay, "Understanding,"[7] offered approaches and orientations that guided my research and my developing clinical practice of attunement. I began thinking about attunement as reflective attention to the actual circumstances of clinical ethics (and research), including the relationships within those circumstances and an awareness of my own actions in light of the power inherent in my roles (whether as clinician or as researcher). That last point is important because clinical ethics consultation – like research – is an inherently and unavoidably social human engagement and, as both Zaner and Bourdieu explicitly say, such activities include potential violence, dominance, distortion that occurs in often asymmetrical social settings. For those on the side of the asymmetry that exhibits more power, the moral experience of such deeply social communication and engagements creates responsibilities for the consultant or the researcher involved.

In that light, regarding the moral engagement of the ethics consultant (or the researcher), the work of my teacher, Mark Bliton, resonated deeply. I took from Bliton's efforts the question of how to actually *ask* about what matters to people and to *listen* in ways that might help them – and help me – as the ethics consultant – to understand the moral concerns and values at stake. Bliton's essay, "Maternal-Fetal Surgery and the 'Profoundest Question in Ethics'"[8] helped me consider the clinical ethicists' responsibility for attending to and responding to what is most relevant to those with whom we are engaged – even when doing so creates risks to ourselves (our self-understandings, our taken-for-granted commitments and values, including those about our role). It is the recognition of these risks inherent in clinical ethics consultation that raises considerations of attunement – what it means and how one practices it in clinical ethics work.

The *rigor* of attunement comes from being available *in* sharing, even temporarily, the questions and circumstances of those for whom such questions are vitally important and sometimes deeply disruptive. Like Wolff's Surrenderer, like Schutz's Stranger, and like the self-reflective moral agents found in Frolic and Ofstad, for the responsible ethicist or reflexive researcher, attunement requires the willingness to engage crucial questions with others with an openness and attention to what matters to them, a recognition of and willingness to suspend one's commitments to their own assumptions, and a practiced, self-reflective awareness of the interaction *as it is occurring.* Bliton's "The Profoundest Question," Bourdieu's "Understanding," and Zaner's "Phenomenology and the Clinical Event" each wrestle with these elements of practice and *method,* and thus help illustrate the importance of attunement to responsible clinical ethics work.

As noted in previous chapters, stories about experiences can illustrate the key elements of clinical ethics practice, and the story that follows represents an example of attunement. "Me and the Moms" is broken into sections that highlight crucial aspects for attunement, followed by a more thorough exploration of Zaner, Bourdieu, and Bliton. The back-and-forth between experiences and reflections is intended to show the challenges in preparation and openness, in affiliation and of listening-and-telling, and of attending to one's own commitments and responses while in the middle of paying careful attention to others in conversation.

### Me and the MOMS: ***Tuesday***

He was a fluttering bird, circling the carved marble of her shoulders. Their gazes pinned me to the doorway while I blinked at them, surrounded by the soft yellow wallpaper of the conference room. I gulped down my awkwardness and tried to smile – kindly, but not too brightly: this was not a social call and not a cheerful moment.

They didn't smile back. They just looked at me with a mild curiosity and resignation. It wasn't hostile, and I knew better than to take it for rudeness, but it was a clue. Everyone I'd met with in this room before had mustered a smile – however wan – or a tilt of the head indicating interest. This was different and, this time, I was alone.

"Hi there. My name is Virginia Bartlett. I'm with the Clinical Ethics Service. May I come in?"

They nodded and the line of her mouth got the faintest bit tighter, as if she wished she could have said "No" but knew better than to try. I walked forward with a thank you and turned to shut the door behind me carefully. I used the moment of my averted face to remind myself I had been in these conversations before. I knew the flow, the orientations and openness I needed to hold; that my mentor would not have me doing this on my own if he didn't trust that I could do it. I visualized the preparatory notes I had written, typed, read aloud, read again, practically memorized in case I got stuck in the middle of the consultation conversation. It hadn't begun, really, and I was already calling to mind the black ink:

*Mental notes for prenatal surgery consults – Reminders:*

- *This is important for them in ways that are impossible for me to understand.*
- *Its ok for the "family face" to be presented and maintained. Armor serves a purpose.*
- *I have to risk misunderstanding in profound ways. And try to understand.*

I turned to the table where they sat, small and round, bringing us a little closer than strangers normally sit. His eyes got a little brighter, showing a shade more interest as I settled my body into the vinyl padding of the institutional chairs. I smiled a little more openly now, with my mind running to the first process question on the list.

"It's Sally, right? And Theodore – oh, you go by Theo? Ok. has anyone with the MOMS study told you why you're talking with someone from Ethics today?"

"Not really." Her voice was quieter than I expected, and flat. Warning bells in my head: was this what I was going to face the whole conversation? My anxiety catastrophized immediately to all the ways I might mess this up, fear that I wasn't up for the work, for helping this couple. My heart sank, until her husband piped up.

"We figured it was part of the informed consent, right hon? That's what you thought? That this was about the research part of the study?" He turned his head toward mine, as he gave her shoulder a quick side-squeeze. "Sally did her medical residency here a few years ago, so she knows all this stuff more than me."

I nodded and smiled. "I think I heard from Tori, the research nurse, that you had some associations here. And you're right – having an ethics consultation *is* part of the research protocol … but it's actually for you all more than for the protocol's sake. I'm here to help you think about this decision, and to help you imagine what might happen over the next few days and months."

I saw Sally's eyebrow go up, again, just slightly. She was holding herself in tight check – but I was watching with a hawk's attention to shadow, light, movement. I continued, "This is a complicated decision that you'll probably be thinking about for a long time to come. I'm not here to judge or evaluate – there aren't right or wrong answers here. But my job is to ask some of the difficult questions, to ask some of the "why?" questions that I've learned people think about, but sometimes have a hard time saying out loud."

Sally and Theo nodded their agreement, or at least their willingness. Relieved, I plowed forward: "It would help me understand some of what you're thinking if you could tell me how you learned about the spina bifida diagnosis."

Their confusion at the question was evident in the half-beat of silence that followed. My brain flashed up the grounding and orienting frames to set-up the questions:

*One thing I've learned in talking with people is that one of the key moments for people, for their moral experience is when they get the diagnosis of spina bifida.*

- *When did you learn of diagnosis? From whom? What did they tell you about prognosis?*
- *What next? When did you decide to contact MOMS?*

I didn't get a chance to reframe or ask any of those supplementing or clarifying questions before Sally suddenly opened up, launching into the facts. I heard her medical training structure every syllable of her recitation:

"We got the diagnosis after an abnormal quad-screen and went in for a level two ultrasound at the OB's office. They told us the lesion on his back was L5/S1, but that there was little or no hydrocephalus. He did show signs of Chiari II malformation as well. That's it. Our high-risk OB told us about the MOMS trial and we started looking into the prenatal surgery option immediately."

Theo nodded, his eye's never leaving Sally's face – looking for something? I couldn't tell, and I was looking too. Sally laughed a short chuckle as she went on.

"I began researching, reading everything I could. I emailed everyone and anyone I knew who might know something about it. I spoke to three women who had come here before to consider the trial. Two enrolled, one didn't. They all told me it was a great experience, and the two who enrolled told me they were happy they had signed up. They both spoke highly of the care they got – even though one got the prenatal surgery and one got randomized to the post-natal repair."

Her voice stopped suddenly, like she almost couldn't bear to say those words. I made a quiet "mmmhmmm" sound and then let the silence sit for a moment – waiting to see if anything else would emerge. When Theo looked at me again, expectantly, I went onward.

"What have you been thinking about between the diagnosis and getting here to Vanderbilt? Do you find yourself leaning towards enrolling in the trial, or looking for more information?"

There! That was close to the mark of how to pose the question, to open it up. I wasn't trying to remember a script, but I had learned phrasing and invitations that worked before …

Theo jumped into answer: "Oh, we're both interested in pre-natal surgery! If you have a way to enroll us right now, and get us into the prenatal group, sign us up!"

He flashed a charming grin and a little chuckle, but his eyes were scanning mine for a possibility. I blinked and Sally, in her near monotone, interjected, "I feel like I have a good grasp on the information. I mean, we know as much as we need to know about the prenatal surgery and the trial. We want to do it."

"Why?"

The question slipped out quietly before I could frame it or present it. Those three letters were stark in their brevity and felt like I made a demand, rather than an invitation. I cringed, but Sally didn't react – just answered the question, as if barked at her by an attending physician in her residency.

"I just, we just think it would be the best thing we can do for our son. The chance of reducing the need for a shunt is the primary motivation, really. I've read that it seems to help children with lesions levels similar to Baby Theo's. The shunt rate for his lesion level is around 75% and if surgery can reduce that risk, it will be worth all the rest, all the other risks."

This last bit came out with the slightest catch in her voice. I wondered if I'd really heard it – but I saw Theo's fingers tighten briefly on her shoulder and knew it was real. And I knew it was important to drill down. I hoped. I saw an opening, perhaps …

***Please tell me about your experience since you've been here: What have you learned?*** *[Sometimes people get different information here than from their local physicians – experience, equipment, etc. sometime provide more detailed information]*

"Can you tell me what you've learned about the risks? From your own research and from meeting with the doctors here?" I hoped for … I don't know what. Some affect? Some engagement? I got a report given by rote – it felt memorized, whether for their comfort or to demonstrate that they had, indeed, read the fine print.

"We talked to the NICU team about how they handle prematurity. We know the children's hospital here is amazing, if Baby Theo needed it for some reason." Theo's confidence bordered on nonchalance, as if he didn't really believe their baby could need the NICU.

"I'm not worried about the risks to myself, if that's what you're asking," said Sally. "I know these are good doctors – and I did train here. They'll take care of me. and I'm in really good health. I know the really serious risks *are* risks, but they're rare. I know about – and I worry about – prematurity, but I'm convinced – we both are – that the potential benefits of prenatal surgery outweigh those risks." She looked at the wall behind me during her recitation with such focus that I had to resist the urge to glance that way.

Theo met and held my gaze for a moment and said "We've been talking about all these things, almost every day. On the phone, over email. We've just decided that the risks outweigh the benefits. We want prenatal surgery." Sally looked at me, cautiously, checking to see if I'd heard them.

I had heard. But I had also heard something else – a hidden mantra – a calm firmness from Theo that felt different from Sally's rote recitation. There was something there that needed air. I skipped ahead in my mental notes – hoping I was following the trail of problems, the puzzles of these two.

*What are you imagining will be the outcome:*

- *if you enroll? if you get prenatal surgery? if you get post-natal surgery?*
- *if you go home? Why not just go home and take care of yourself and the rest of your pregnancy? It is an equally acceptable moral choice to go home.*

I hesitated, and shifted in my seat, leaning forward a little. "You know, as I said at the beginning, that one of my jobs is to help you imagine possible outcomes and to think about as many things as possible beforehand. Can we do that? Together?" They nodded, together, Sally's gaze wary, Theo's curious.

"Okay. It sounds like you're imagining having the prenatal surgery, and imagining that it all goes well, that it is beneficial for your baby."

They both kind of grinned at each other, like I had discovered their secret, that they knew was transparent but weren't going to mention otherwise. "Yeah, that's true," said Theo, and I saw Sally reach her left hand up to squeeze his fingers still draped over her shoulder. I hated the words that were about to come out of my mouth, but I couldn't not say them.

"I want you to imagine that you have the prenatal surgery, but that it is not successful. That the baby comes under 30 weeks and you two have a severely premature infant with the multiple problems from the spina bifida as well. Or that this baby dies. That little Theo doesn't make it through surgery or survive such a pre-term delivery." I glued my eyes to their faces. "Can you imagine what your thoughts might be? Or your responses? Because these are real risks. They happen to real people."

They looked at each other and Sally dropped her hand to her lap again. "I don't think we would blame ourselves or feel bad about our decision. I think we'd know that we tried to do everything we could to help our child."

Theo nodded fervently, "We will be okay with whatever happens. We would be sad, of course, if we lost our son, but we would be okay. We'd know we had made the best decision we could with the information we had, with the choices facing us. In the end, that's all you can do, right? Decisions based on what you know."

Sally sighed, "We are sure we want the surgery. And we know God will take care of us."

Part of my mind had been wandering through my preparatory list of questions – trying to connect to something in this near impenetrable commitment to going forward with prenatal surgery. There seemed to be no other option, no other possibility in their world. I wondered if it was coming from a deep faith place – that was a motivation, my teachers and I had learned, for many women and their partners. But when faith was the motivator, it tended to be a more public, a more evangelical kind of faith, which appeared much earlier in their stories as a primary fact and framework. I hadn't gotten any sense of that kind of religious commitment, but maybe I'd missed it in my anxiety about this first solo consultation.

"Sally, could you tell me more about God taking care of you? A lot of the people we speak to talk about their faith or God's will – could you talk about that some more?" It was a long moment of her looking at me in silence. I wondered if I'd broken the conversation. Had I crossed a line or opened an avenue she wouldn't or couldn't walk?

She shook her head a quick second and shrugged. "I don't believe it's God's will in the sense of already decided – I don't believe things happen just because God decides or that God reaches down to intervene. Humans decide and have to act. But I believe in God's love and I know God will care for us."

Theo sat silent, looking at his wife as she talked about faith – her faith? Their faith? I couldn't tell. Something felt off and I risked the question: "Is this something you two have talked about? Are these beliefs you share?"

Theo nodded enthusiastically, and I was reminded again of a bird aflutter – a weird association for a large, strong-looking man. "Oh yes, we both have strong faith and I know we'll be able to handle whatever happens. Especially with our families praying for us too. They're lifting us up, and are ready to help, whatever we decide to do. All four parents are actually here, in town with us, and Sally's mom will stay with her if we get the prenatal surgery. She's a nurse, too, so she can help with both Sally and baby." He grinned again at some vision of the future where all of this worked out beautifully.

No lack of belief or faith there, although I still sensed some disconnect between them and their commitments. Yet, I'd heard the opening in Theo's comments to get back to imagining the what ifs – the possibilizing beyond the imagined ideal.

"Having Sally's mom here would be great if you all get the prenatal surgery. I also wonder if you can imagine with me: how would you feel if you got randomized to the post-natal surgery. This is a randomized controlled trial, so we have no idea which way things will go until we enter everything into the computer and the machine up at George Washington, the coordination site, gives us the randomization. Would you all be happy if you got the post-natal surgery?"

I cringed as the last words came out before I could stop them. Happy was not the right register, the right tenor for the question I was after. Sally's eyebrow climbed to the ceiling as she said, "Well, no. We won't be happy. We do want the prenatal surgery. That's what we're hoping for because we think it will help."

I kept my gaze as open and inviting as I could, hoping she would say more. She continued, "But we also want to participate to help with the research. Research on spina bifida has helped children survive longer and with better outcomes. And this is part of that research, so in the end, if we get post-natal surgery, we'll be ok."

I tried to think of how to move to other questions, other angles to consider, but Sally opened the door herself. "Besides, at least we're still getting the best care for me and the baby. The neurosurgeons here will close Baby Theo's spine either way."

I heard it again, the commitment to the trial being therapeutic instead of research. I pushed, again, and told them I was pushing on the idea of it helping. "This trial is not designed to help your baby. It is designed to look at two groups and compare them." I heard my teacher, Mark's, voice inside my head, hammering on the gravity of the point: the words came out almost verbatim from my mental notes: "and with two groups, if the surgery turns out not to be beneficial, then we have protected one group of women from harm."

They pushed back too, Theo insisting: "We know all that! We really do! But we're still convinced we can get the best care through the trial."

I tried one more time – I felt like I had to, like there was something else there, just below what they were willing, or able, to share. I wanted to try to open up that space one more time.

"I hear you. I do. But I just have to make sure you know – really – that you can still get the best care here even without enrolling in the trial. You can go home for the next few months, take care of the pregnancy and yourselves, come back here to have this team do the delivery and spina bifida repair. I just want to emphasize that would be a perfectly moral choice, perfectly acceptable way of "doing something" for your baby – without taking all these risks to the baby, and to you, Sally."

As I spoke, their heads shook back and forth, rejecting that possibility. "No, we know all that, but really," said Theo, "we feel like this is what we want to do. We want to be a part of it."

We looked at each other for a quiet moment while my mind ran rapid fire over possible questions, darting through flashbacks of conversations with other women considering MOMS trial enrollment. I kept coming back to my reminder, my note to self, that it's okay for the family face to be maintained. They were so adamant about joining the study, so insistent about this possibly reducing the need for a shunt that pushing harder, that piercing the armor of their story didn't seem likely to elicit a different understanding, and might cross the line into a kind of harm. Even though this conversation had been just 45 minutes, I chose to close it down. I wasn't sure how I could – or why I should – reframe the same things I'd already asked.

After the eternity of that moment, I took a breath "I hear you. And thank you for thinking out loud with me. Are there any questions you have for me? Questions I can answer, or I could find out who to ask for answers?"

Sally sighed (with relief? I wondered), "No, thank you. We've done so much research already and talked to everyone we need here."

Theo tilted his head to one side, looking at me quizzically. "So, what is your part in all of this? Are you part of the trial?"

I was a little stunned. It was as if he just now realized he could ask me why they had to talk to me in the first place. Maybe it was. Maybe they hadn't heard anything of what I said when I introduced myself, that I was just another face interrogating them, another gate they had to get through before they could enroll and get the pre-natal surgery they were sure would help their son.

I sighed inside and smiled a little when I answered, "Yes, my mentor and I usually talk with potential participants but he's out of town, so it's just me today." I took the moment to try to explain again. "The ethics part of this trial is important – to help people think about their choices and decision in as many ways as possible. I've talked to about twenty families so far, but my mentor has talked with nearly everyone – for this trial, and in the early elective surgery series. We try to see what people are thinking about. To help them think out loud. It's not to evaluate their thinking, but to understand, and to help them understand their own thought processes."

Theo nodded as he listened, mulling it over, but I could see Sally was getting a bit of a glazed look in her eyes. I met her gaze and held it for a moment: "One of my concerns is that after the diagnosis, which is so devastating for many people, the urge to do something is really strong. Especially for the mothers. I just want to make sure you don't feel pressured into taking these risks when you don't have to …" Sally looked at me and gave a curt nod: "I can see that."

I continued, "That's part of why I try to emphasize the risks. That they are real. And that it is perfectly acceptable to go home and just come back for the delivery." She shook her head, harder this time. "No. no, we talked about this, but we've decided this is what we want to do."

I nodded and smiled at them. "Alright then, these are all the questions I have. Thank you so much for sharing and talking with me. We'll meet again with the whole team in the morning, so if you do discover any questions, you'll let me know and we can talk then."

We all stood, and I watched as Theo gathered their things: a backpack, her shoulder bag. She moved carefully toward the door I held open, and we walked toward the research office and their checkout and review of the plans for tomorrow.

I couldn't shake my uneasiness, a sickly fear that I had missed something, had failed them. I saw her walking beside me – so contained – not like a statue after all. But a bridge cable, buffeted in high winds, its steel fibers twisting tighter inward, lest they snap, and everything crashes down.

### *Uncanny Circumstances Require Extraordinary Attention*

This first solo consult was disconcerting and even disorienting. I was *ready* and yet struggled throughout to understand if my "ready" was enough for their needs. I recognized that preparation and invitation were necessary on my end, but that did not mean they would engage or respond to the invitation. The challenge was trying to listen for and hear their concerns or questions – even the ones they couldn't or wouldn't speak out loud. And the risk of focusing such attention on another human being is that it can feel intrusive, be challenging. We don't usually talk about things that matter so deeply in typical day-to-day conversations – we continue onward, using our everyday, taken-for-granted recipes for making sense of our worlds and the actions of others in our worlds. To question, especially to deliberately probe the meanings and values behind another's words and actions risks violation – of that person's understandings, commitments, and sense of safety or surety. It is the risk and the requirement of the Stranger's engagement.

Even if necessary, however, such engagement might also put into question the consultant's understandings, commitments, and sense of safety or surety. The risk to the participants in clinical ethics consultation – including the ethics consultant – is part of what sets these conversations and encounters apart from the ordinary. The conversation, when genuine, can move them into unspoken, and even uncanny, meanings and requires an extraordinary attention: an attunement. In the circumstances that prompt a clinical ethics consultation – like the MOMS trial situation described here – the demand is for preparation and attention to the usual and expected concerns like those outlined in my Mental Notes, *and* sensitivity to the unique and unexpected. Even with my preparation and previous experiences, I found myself uncertain of how to understand Sally's reticence, especial in contrast to Theo's insouciant confidence, Even more challenging, I was hesitant to touch, to push too hard on the unspoken disconnect in how they talked about their faith in their decision-making. Something seemed to matter, just below the surface, deliberately out of reach.

The challenge illustrated here is one that is common, if not always acknowledged, in clinical ethics consultation: that even with necessary preparation, practiced attention, and self-reflective openness, it is not always clear if the consultation conversation is sufficient, or adequate to the situation of *these particular participants*. Hence, attunement is a necessary element and is an ongoing activity in clinical ethics practice. Further, these practices of attunement by the clinical ethics consultant may require their own kind attention and extraordinary conversation – before, during, or after the consultation experience. In my consultation with Sally and Theo, the attunement continued after our initial conversation, as meanings became clearer through conversation with and corroboration by other involved in their care.

### Me and the MOMS: *** Tuesday, Late Afternoon***

Tori, the research nurse, stood halfway in the doorway, waving goodbye and admonishing Sally and Theo to rest up before tomorrow. I could hear their murmured responses fading down the hall as Tori slipped the rest of herself back inside the research office and shut the door behind her. I tried not to fidget and squirm as I sat waiting, but I felt unreleased tension burbling through my body, my mind bouncing back through my conversations with the couple that just left. I felt myself preparing for the question I knew Tori would ask – because it's the question she always asks: an utterly banal and fully loaded "Well, how did it go?" Today I was the one who had to answer, to capture and reflect and report on the ethics conversation, and she was aware of that too. She added more questions before I could answer the first. "This was your first one all by yourself, right? How are you doing?"

The unexpectedness of being asked about myself spurred a nervous laugh and I shook my head. "Still working on figuring all those out." Tori smiled as she walked over to sit beside Sue, the social worker, while we waited for the surgeon to join us. At the end of the second day, after the potential MOMS trial participant and her support person had met with the physicians, the surgeons, the NICU team, social work, Tori, and ethics, everyone on the team gathered to discuss. Each team member was expected to share their impressions about whether the pregnant woman met the study's inclusion criteria, didn't have any of the exclusion criteria, and didn't trigger anyone's sixth sense about coercion, instability, or other factors that might make them higher risk – for themselves and the study. Today, I was the one speaking for the ethics portion of the MOMS evaluation.

While we waited for the surgeon, I talked to Tori, who had become a friend, of sorts, through my training, through previous MOMS trial consultations and surgery observations. "I don't know Tori. I've been thinking through since I finished the conversation with them. It was tough. In part because it was my first time holding that conversation alone – for sure. But I think I did well, and it wasn't hard just because Mark wasn't here. Sally and Theo and I talked about and talked through all the things that normally come up – or that Mark and I bring up – when we have had these conversations before. I asked for their story from diagnosis to getting here. We clarified and went over the risks, the research aspect and randomization. I pushed on all the possibilities – prenatal and postnatal surgery, things going well or something catastrophic happening. I asked about religious motivations when she started talking about God watching over them. But I don't feel like the consult ever opened up."

Tori nodded and I paused, chewing on my lower lip as I thought. She gestured for me to keep talking and I went on. "It felt rehearsed. Like a performance piece, more than a conversation. Theo was more open than Sally was – more engaged, paying more attention to the questions and the way the conversation was going, but also watching her, seeing how she was doing. He really didn't speak as much."

Both Tori and Sue nodded and looked at each other, with some shared understanding – as if they'd already discussed something like what I was saying. I sighed and shrugged. "I'm worried that I missed something. Sally did most of the talking, but I really got the sense she was saying what she had learned she had to say, what she was expected to say. She had thought about all the issues, that was obvious. She'd done all her homework, had educated herself about the MOMS trial, about the prenatal procedure. But it felt like I was getting a report, even a sales-pitch 'See we've ticked all the boxes! We can prove we know the risks.'" But I didn't get a sense that she really understood whether or not any of them were about her – that she was at risk and she didn't have to be. I don't know. After nearly an hour, I don't think I was getting anywhere close to what she was actually thinking about. Except that she says she wants the prenatal surgery."

Sue smiled, but it was a grim sort of smile: not quite cynical, but unpleasantly unsurprised. "You didn't miss anything, honey. That was spot on, and we've all had the same experience. She's wrapped super tight about all of this and has been since she got here. She's not letting anyone in. And her husband – for all he looks like he's lumberjack tough – he's the one with the nervous excitement – like it's all *just got to* work out fine."

Tori nodded too, and added, "As soon as Sally found out about the spina bifida, she started emailing and calling everyone she could. Anyone who was associated with Vanderbilt or the MOMS trial central office up at George Washington. She was trying to see if there was a way she could just get the prenatal surgery – to skip the trial and randomization. She wanted to do the prenatal surgery as soon as possible because she'd heard or read that earlier was better – and she was 17 weeks gestation when she found out."

I felt my eyebrow rise and I willed it back down, trying to keep my face neutral and impassive, even if my inner voice was getting huffy and sputtering at the idea of someone trying to use connections to skip the trial protocols – to not follow the rules.

In the nanosecond of Tori's catching her breath to continue, I had just about talked myself out of an unfair, uncharitable judgment, when she continued giving me and Sue the backstory. "Sally realized she had to go through the trial to have any chance of getting prenatal surgery – remember, all the centers in the country agreed to a national moratorium on elective or experimental procedures while the trial was running – for just this reason! People – these moms are so desperate to *do something* that they wouldn't enroll in the trial if they could just choose prenatal surgery, but then we still wouldn't have clear evidence of whether the benefits are worth the risks. Anyway, Sally was one of those who wanted to do something and was convinced this would help. So, she agreed to come up for the evaluation and possible enrollment. But *then* she wanted to come that next week – but we already had two women scheduled for evaluation and possible surgery if they enrolled and got randomized to prenatal. She asked and pushed to see if she could "skip ahead" of them and go first. Uh huh … Man oh man: I could hear the panic in her voice."

My uncharitable judgment was feeling more and more justified. Although I resisted the feeling of judgment either way, there it was. I was flat out indignant that someone would try to jump ahead of two other women in the same circumstance – who were also probably panicked and heartbroken. How could Sally do that? How could anyone? I squirmed again, physically uncomfortable with this information and the direction my thoughts were taking. I closed my lips to not speak even accidently. I remembered her tight eyes and still body and thought, how could she not? Still, I was relieved that I had not known this part of the story before I talked to them. I don't know what I would have done, walking in with those heavy criticisms in my mind and heart. It would have been hard to maintain sympathy – which I did feel for them – if I'd heard all her answers and felt her reserve through the lens of judging her for trying to bump other people out of line, to get her child treated first.

Tori continued, "Sally called and talked to the folks at GW again, and they offered that if she really wanted to, she could go up to Philadelphia, to one of the other trial centers. But she and Theo decided to wait and come back to Vanderbilt. They seem to have made some peace with the trial and with waiting when they got here. What did you think?"

I pinched my fingers back and forth across my brow bones, trying to loosen the tension headache that was building steadily. "Well, that part of their journey didn't come up in our conversation," I said ruefully. "But it does shine a whole different light on all their jokes about 'Tell them where to sign!' and 'What button do we push?' to get the prenatal surgery. I'm not sure they really accept or believe the possibilities that it might not help. Or not work. Or that they could get postnatal repair."

Sue gave her sardonic half smile again and looked up as the surgeon who would be performing the surgery stuck their head in the door. "Any news? Are we meeting in the morning? She meets all the surgical inclusion criteria, and none of the exclusions – I spoke with the neurosurgery team – they think she looks like a good candidate if she randmonizes to prenatal."

Sue was the one who replied as she sighed, "Well, that's certainly what they want. I had no doubt they'll enroll. It's just a question of if they'll stick with it if they get assigned to the postnatal arm."

The surgeon looked momentarily confused – as if they, too, hadn't considered the possibility of *not* doing the prenatal procedure on this patient. I remembered in a flash: the study obstetrician was also out of town. If Sally went to surgery, it would be one of the first times for this surgeon to be primary for the obstetric part – the C-section opening and hysterotomy. They'd assisted before, but this would be their first time as lead if the surgery was scheduled for this week. More uncharitable thoughts arose: no wonder the surgeon looked so concerned at the thought of a post-natal repair. They'd miss their chance to shine if the randomization went that way.

Tori shook her head and said, "No, I think they're in it, either way. They seem committed to the neurosurgeons here doing the spina bifida repair, whether prenatal or post-natal. Did you get a sense when you talked to them?" She passed the question to me and I felt three pairs of eyes on my face.

"I think they're so committed to the prenatal surgery that they're not really thinking about the postnatal, but they did say they'd get the best care here either way. I think they'll stay in either way. And they noted the altruism angle – helping spina bifida research for the long term. Which doesn't quite outweigh the risks, does it? But they don't seem worried about the risks – kept saying this was the best place for care."

"Great!" the surgeon nearly bounced up and down in their excitement. "So, we'll meet here at 8:30 in the morning? And I'm supposed to read over all the consents with them, right? In case they have any questions? But you all will be there to help too, right?" Tori nodded and the surgeon gave a grin and half salute and whistled down the hall as the door closed behind them.

I had a moment's disconnect, wondering if we were in the same reality: the one where we were offering a fifty-fifty chance at a surgery on Sally's baby – while in utero – to fix a congenital defect that was disabling, but not lethal. And we were only offering a fifty-fifty chance because there was a 5% chance – one in twenty – that the baby could die, or Sally could have serious injury and possibly die. But the surgeon, like Theo, was nearly giddy with enthusiasm about the possibility of prenatal surgery. I shuddered and gave some distracted goodbyes to Sue and Tori as we wrapped up and gathered our things.

And I walked down the hill from the medical center to my car, rewinding and replaying the conversation with Sally and Theo. The one thing I kept pushing on with them was imagining how they would feel if they got the postnatal arm. And that turned out to be the thing that needed pushing. As I walked, I had moments of simple pride and some satisfaction that I'd puzzled it out, that I'd caught the clues and kept probing to understand, to invite them to share their thoughts. But each moment of satisfaction crumbled with the relived recognitions that I kept coming back to it because they wouldn't talk about it, really. They were so convinced of the benefit, so adamant about wanting the trial and wanting to get the prenatal surgery, that it seemed like they hadn't really considered anything else. I pushed because I found myself cringing to think of how they would react if they did get randomized to post-natal surgery. They kept saying they would be ok, just like they kept saying they knew and understood the risks and were ok with those too. But it felt untrue, no matter how sincerely she spoke. And I walked home holding the uncomfortable feeling that I hadn't really gotten to what I needed to help them – that I hadn't been able to help at all – and that even if the chance came by tomorrow, to try once more, I would be hesitant to bring it up again.

### Richard M. Zaner: Attention to the Actual Circumstances at Hand

In both the immediate aftermath of my encounter with Sally and Theo – and with the members of the research team – I struggled to make sense of the taken-for-granted values at play, and to understand the meanings revealed in the extraordinary moments of conversation. Then and now, the challenge is moving between the clinical encounter itself and the process of understanding what all matters for the practice of clinical ethics – in and beyond the particular encounter.

What connects the unique and *sui generis* circumstances (and the unique, actual, biographically, historically situated person consulting) to the broader questions of practice? What gives this story any relevance to another ethics consultant's practice or similar circumstance for another family? One of the most helpful ways to think about it comes from Richard M. Zaner's 1994 essay, "Phenomenology and the Clinical Event."[9] The essay is a clear articulation of how phenomenology can inform and shape the practice of clinical ethics and clinical ethics consultation, and in re-readings through this stage of my own practice, it has a clarity that sings and resonates on deeper levels. It was a struggle to understand at the beginning of my clinical training and practice, without much experience from which to draw, and when attunement seemed such a funny word. I've learned since that the practice of attunement in consultation, the deliberate and intentional focusing of attention to the everyday, can create the extraordinary space for extraordinary communication in the ordinary experiences and encounters with other humans.

Seminar, it turns out, was an exercise in attunement; as were each of my clinical exposures in MICU and NICU. That lightning bolt of discovering or being drawn to something calling for attention, that signals its importance – and demands paying attention to the specific circumstances, the others involved, and one's own actions. It is both a mundane moral endeavor, and, in Zaner's phenomenological practice, a set of rigorous activities aimed at understanding "what's going on?" in a given situation.

*Moral Factors and Situational Definitions*

The starting normative claim from Zaner's work about ethics consultation is that the ethics consultant seeks to identify and remain faithful to significant moral features found in complex layers of contexts, values, and persons found in clinical encounters. Zaner's concern is the inquiry through which we learn by trying to identify and possibly understand certain themes and activities, while reflecting on the changing circumstances of a conversation and the engagement of its participants, and how they can affect meanings and understandings. The first step toward attunement is to discover what matters in *this* circumstance for *these* participants.

For Zaner, clinically presented problems and moral issues, activities and possible outcomes, are context specific and require "a strict focus on the situational definitions of each involved person."[10] Such efforts require discovering and clarifying, not only who is involved and why but also what they understand about the circumstances at hand and what meanings they assign to various features of these circumstances. As Zaner explains,

> to understand the clinical situation, there is nothing for it but to try one's best to get at the concrete ways the participants themselves experience and understand the situations, and endow its various components (objects people, things, relationships) with meanings.[11]

Discovering what matters, probing the questions and claims of others requires the ethicist to be attuned to – sensitized to – the broader circumstances in which participants' stories emerge.

The challenge, and the responsibility, is to be deliberately reflectively attentive – rigorously attuned – to the other who tells me of her experiences, who makes meaning(s) out of her story. As Zaner points out,

> Moral issues are presented for deliberation, decision, and resolution solely within the context of their actual occurrence. To find out and understand what's going on in any clinical event – what's troubling the people, what's on their minds, and thus to know what has to be addressed and how, requires cautious attentive probing to the ongoing discourse, conduct, the setting, and other matters presented as constituting a particular context.[12]

Ethics consultation often involves helping people make sense of their experiences in the midst of complex familial, clinical, or professional relationships. The attunement also includes creating a deliberate openness to as many available meanings, ambiguities, and uncertainties in the experiences as possible, as Zaner reflects in a later essay:

> The people whom I met in these clinical encounters sought not only to tell me and others what they were going through, with all their uncertainties and ambiguities, but wanted me to listen while at the same time helping them assimilate their sense of themselves and their beliefs.[13]

Because any given consultation may include multiple others, "a veritable chorus (sometimes a riot) of voices, each anxious to be heard,"[14] the attunement is a resolutely active and engaged practice – an opening and learning rather than a reducing, simplifying, and having heard already.

### Acts of Affiliation

The complexity of the chorus of voices and multivalent meanings in clinical encounters – or research encounters – makes the clinical ethics consultant's job, according to Zaner, part detective work, part enablement and empowerment. He describes the task as helping participants,

> Identify what is at issue for each person, to help each become alert to and consider their respective moral frameworks; to help deliberate, weigh, and imaginatively probe the available options that are most reasonable and fitting with those respective frameworks; and to help each attain clarity about the "stakes" so as to enable them to live with the outcomes or aftermaths of needed decisions.[15]

This description of Zaner's resonated with me years ago as I was conducting my dissertation interviews and participating in and leading MOMS trial ethics consultations, and it resonates now, reflecting on my practice, years later. The resonance is in the openness: attunement is a less a procedural prescription and more an orientation toward practice. Zaner emphasizes a deliberate suspension of typical understandings, a way to direct attention to the particular issues at hand – similar to the practices and orientation of the Stranger and the Surrenderer.

The deliberate shift of attention allows for the careful identification of the possibilities of and effects of uncertainty, error, and deception on understanding – imagining and "possibilizing" the different understandings, decisions, and actions that may emerge.[16] These accounts of careful and specific attention to the circumstances at hand create the possibility for the ethics consultant to "place oneself in the lived experience of the patient" – the possibility of what Zaner also calls "affiliation." Affiliation is an orientation and effort toward "understanding that person's circumstance from her own perspective, as she lives and understands it – disclosed contextually through her discourse, paralinguistic features, and bodily demeanor."[17] This practice of affiliation has deep parallels, as I develop below, to Pierre Bourdieu's concerns for a reflexive method of sociology, and affiliation highlights the importance of shared talking and listening as the method for and access to such understanding. The lesson from Zaner is that to practice such talking and listening – and to reflect on the circumstances in which such talking and listening emerge – "is to learn about moral life from the clinical circumstances of those who actually face difficult circumstances."[18]

This phase of attunement, attending to what matters in the particular and actual circumstances, as presented by (and learned from the person directly involved, the person for whom some concern is at stake) requires *being with* the other in their concern, in their circumstance as much as can be. Attention to the circumstances, then, is deeply connected to and dependent on the idea of affiliation with the other person, and it is here that Pierre Bourdieu's work on interviewing in sociological research explicates performative interactions in conversation that are resonant, generative, and crucially relevant to clinical ethics work.

## Me and the MOMS: ***Wednesday Morning***

It was a full house for the drama of the moment. I'd joined Tori and Sue in the conference room before Sally and Theo walked in, flanked by Sally's parents and Theo's mom. I joined in the introductions and smiles. It was a weirdly social interaction in a medicalized setting for a scientific research project. These discordances were both evident to all those involved and likewise actively ignored, even when the surgeon came in and joined the chatter. Everything is fine, nothing more to see here …

Everyone settled into seats: the parents on the couch in the back of the room; Tori, Sue, the surgeon, and me at the table with Sally and Theo. I scanned faces and bodies, taking note of the near nonchalance of the surgeon's posture and Sally's hands, tightly gripped in her lap, Theo's arm lurking across the back of her chair – ready to surround her shoulders if needed. Sue watched speculatively – the calm and problem-solving bent to her training an observation post for the emotions at play. Tori was ready for business, getting stacks of paper into twin piles – one for the family, one for the study files.

"Do you have any questions for Sally and Theo before we begin?" Tori's question startled me into a smile, and I focused on the faces in front of me. I was going to have to ask again.

"Ah … sure. So, from our conversation yesterday, you were both pretty clear you wanted to enroll …"

They nodded in agreement and looked at each other – Theo with an excited grin, Sally with an unblinking stare. I continued. "We did talk about many possibilities – risks and harms, and also getting assigned to the post-natal arm. Are you still willing to accept either arm of the trial?"

I had an uncomfortable moment of feeling like a cleric, seeking the solemn promises of a wedding vow, searching for avowals of commitment. Theo's buoyant attempt at humor lifted that veil.

"We do! But if there's any way to trick the computer toward prenatal surgery …" Everyone chucked as his voice trailed off suggestively. I felt a clenched fist in my gut – repeated jabs: they still don't get it – they still don't know – they are *ignoring* the danger. I have failed: a twisting mantra, just below my throat.

Tori handed around copies of the consent form for them to read with her and the surgeon before signing – two copies each. I blinked and swallowed hard when Theo commented on the size of it. I tried again, indirectly: "The form is big because it goes over the risks in detail – and lots of people have new questions when they read it. Please ask if you do."

They didn't. They nodded through Tori's and the surgeon's explanations and signed every page with an urgency to be done. Tori thanked them and excused herself from the table, turning to the computer on the wall. She carefully entered the data and measurements from Sally's medical exams, each inclusion or exclusion criteria leaving a green check-mark on the screen. Everyone watched every keystroke and click of the mouse – communicating all their hopes to an unseen randomization algorithm in the computer up at the MOMS Study center.

In a long 30 seconds, held breaths erupted when the assignment was prenatal surgery. Theo's stadium volume "Whoohooo!" startled Tori out of her chair and he almost didn't seem to see Sally's gasping sob break into flowing tears. Tori and I looked at her and she choked out, "It's just joy. I'm crying for joy. I'm so happy, so relieved." I hoped my face didn't show my skepticism as her husband kissed her cheek before turning to hug and high-five her dad.

I scoured the rest of the crowd and saw teary mothers on the couch and Sally's dad talking excitedly with Theo. Sally's mom, with her weepy grin, kept saying "Sally just comes from an emotional family," as if offering an apology to Tori and me.

I was torn between relief for them and that lurking apprehension because they clearly could only see success, and I had learned that term is defined differently by the study team and by the parents post-surgery. I stuffed down and silenced an ugly realization that part of me had hoped they would get post-natal: karmic justice after their efforts to jump ahead of others. With a stab of shame, I realized I'd slipped into that uncomfortable reverie while everyone chattered and hugged and now the quiet was returning.

Everyone stood around the room, grins and tears – happy tears! – being wiped gently away. Theo's mom suddenly spoke up and waved everyone close with her hands. "We should have a prayer and give thanks to God for this blessing! C'mon now!" and she reached for my hand and held me in the circle before I could back away or demure. She directed Sally's mom to start the prayer and then looked expectantly to Sally's dad when his wife stood silent and clearly taken aback. I stifled a bemused observation that not everyone seemed moved to spontaneous halle-lujah. Sally's dad came through before things got too awkward and made a quiet little prayer of thanksgiving for the children, for Baby Theo, for all the blessed people at Vanderbilt, and for this opportunity to care for this beloved baby, perfect child of God. I bowed my head with all the rest, wondering as they all murmured Amens.

### *Pierre Bourdieu: Communication with the Other and Shared Meaning-Making*

Each phase of my encounter with Sally and Theo – and with their research team – and later, their families, revealed new insights into what mattered and what they faced in this decision to enroll in the MOMS trial. I prepared for this encounter by reading, talking with my mentor, practicing and participating in other consultations, and I approached with the kind of open-ness and affiliation described by Zaner. Yet in the actual situations, I discovered commitments I didn't know I carried, and expectations I wasn't fully aware of until they were unmet. I found myself uncertain in the face of Sally's rigid control and skeptical of Theo's efforts to charm his way out of engaging with the questions at hand. I both wanted to push them into facing what I understood to be the key moral questions of this kind of situation, and I didn't want to push them into something beyond what they chose to engage. To think about walking the line between inviting and pushing, between eliciting and enforcing engagement, I found helpful frames in Zaner's affiliation and engaging with the questions *of those with something at stake.* I also found Pierre Bourdieu's idea of *understanding* to be a guiding and grounding theme to make sense of my encounters with Sally and Theo (and with others since that first consultation).

In his 1999 article, "Understanding," Bourdieu explores mutual understanding as generated by way of deliberate, informed non-violent communication between researcher/interviewer and participant/interviewee. In reflecting back on these clinical encounters and how I made sense of them, I found resonances among Bourdieu and other thinkers I had read and studied. Like Frolic, Bourdieu insists on a practice of self-reflection and awareness of one's own commitments. He combines this with preparation and methodical attention to the others with whom one is engaging, as necessary before, during, and after the research encounter. As with Wolff's surrender-to, Bourdieu's practice allows for the possibility of shared meaning and understanding.

Bourdieu is explicit that such understandings develop within a clear acknowledgement that the research relationship is a social relationship (just as Zaner and others have emphasized that the clinical ethics encounter is an inherently social and hence unavoidably moral relationship). Bourdieu resists getting caught by disciplinary commitments informed by reductive methodologies which claim that scientific rigor will prevent social and subjective influence. His work instead acknowledges the inescapably social nature of research and works to develop and articulate a "reflex reflexivity" based on a craft – similar to the attunement in clinical ethics work – that can account for and respond to those social and subjective influences.

In "Understanding," Bourdieu both describes and demonstrates what he calls "the sociological "feel" or "eye" that allows one to perceive or monitor, *on the spot* as the interview is actually taking place, the effects of the social structure within which it is occurring."[19] The social scientist, the interviewer, has to be aware of and responsible "to discover and master as completely as possible the nature of its inevitable acts of construction and the equally inevitable effects those acts produce."[20] In practical terms, this means I have to work deliberately to understand of my own presuppositions. I have to know what they are and the work they do in my thinking, because they inevitably construct and shape how I examine, probe, and understand others' presuppositions in an interview, or in my case an ethics conversation.

Presuppositions, especially when un-examined, can be powerful and can wield great effect in shaping the interview and the research relationship. One real concern arises in the inherent risks of violence and the exertion of power in communication. For Bourdieu, the interviewer thus has to account for their presuppositions – and more. The interviewer is also responsible for ferreting out different perceptions about the goal of the interview or conversation, about the research relationship, and what each participant brings to the interaction regarding language, symbolic, and social goods. With awareness of these differences – and of the researcher's presuppositions and commitments – Bourdieu seeks not to eradicate such social commitments or influences, but "to reduce as much as possible symbolic violence exerted through the relationship."[21] Only by considering, acknowledging, and responding to those influences can the interviewer reduce the possible harms of miscommunication.

Bourdieu is clear that responsibility for this awareness – for developing this "reflex reflexivity" or sociological "feel" – belongs to the researcher before, during, and after the encounters with the interviewee or research subject. What struck so very clearly in my clinical ethics training – and which comes out clearly in my experiences with Sally and Theo is the weight of this responsibility. I felt the same weight in my dissertation interviews, especially the one I described in Chapter 1, "Observations II" with Carin and George Miller.

*Responsibility for Collaborative Construction*

The challenge of fulfilling such a responsibility remains critical for both research and clinical ethics work. In each of those situations, the researcher or the ethics consultant has to know enough about the context, group, issue, etc. to be able to engage with the individual who is presenting their individual self from within that context, group, issue. Or, in language harkening back to Wolff, the interviewer or ethics consultant or investigator has to be able to fully engage with the unique individual in both their individual, historical meanings and their broader, human-writ-large elements. Bourdieu describes setting up a relationship of active and methodical *listening* ...

> (that) combines a total availability to the person being questioned, submission to the singularity of a particular life history – which can lead, by a kind of more or less controlled imitation, to adopting the interviewee's language, views, feelings, and thoughts – with methodical construction founded on the knowledge of the objective conditions common to an entire social category.[22]

The aim is joining the interviewee in their understanding by collaboration in the construction of that understanding and its meaning(s). Similar to Zaner's emphasis on affiliation, Bourdieu argues collaborative construction is more generative if those involved – interviewer and interviewee – "can appropriate the inquiry for themselves and become its subject" – i.e., if they are both trying to discover "what's going on?" or "figure out" what matters together.

The work of collaboration, however, depends on the social relationship and commitment to share understanding, and, per Bourdieu, success is not guaranteed by formula or structure. This may be one of the most crucial recognitions and lessons from Bourdieu and one of the most difficult aspects of my clinical ethics training – and indeed, ongoing practice. Even if all the conditions are created for openness, communication, mitigation of communicative violence, and possible understanding – *understanding may not happen*. Bourdieu's critical importance to the practical elements of clinical ethics is this reminder that the interviewer is responsible for both creating those conditions *and is still responsible* even if they do not lead to the hoped-for clarity and understanding. No algorithm, decision-tree, four box-method, or interview questionnaire will be sufficient for a given situation, though the work of preparing them may be necessary in order for the interviewer (or ethics consultant) to operate carefully, deliberately, responsibly within the context of the conversation. Doing so requires both knowing something about the situation and question at hand – and being explicit and clear and honest and humble about what is not known.

Acknowledging the ambiguity – the uncertainty – may be the hardest part, especially after years of education and training toward "knowing things" as a positive, a good,[23] a mark of expertise. The deliberate cultivation of a beginner's mind – not just the presentation of oneself as having a beginner's mind – but an actual acceptance of one's unknowing and limitations is hard to build and maintain in a world that wants experts with answers, rather than explorers who discover. Part of what resonated and still resonates so deeply about Bourdieu is the idea of both/and: you have to *know* as much as possible about the subjects, the questions, the persons as you can *so that* you have the possibility of hearing and seeing and learning *what you don't know* when you encounter it.

Helping strangers uncover and articulate what may be taken for granted and deeply relevant in their lives requires – at the same time – maintaining the humility of following these strangers' own expertise in their lives too. So, it requires both a familiarity – and strangeness. In talking with Sally and Theo in the intimacy of our first conversation, and in the carnivalesque performative in the enrollment meeting, I had to make the space, to ask the questions I'd learned to ask ... *and* I had to discover when to stop, when to not ask. In the team conference with Tori and Sue, when I most needed to share what I knew, what I'd heard and learned, I had to acknowledge my uncertainty, my remaining questions and how difficult the encounter had been, even though, seen from a structural or procedural view, it was just like all the others, it met all the requirements. I had provided clinical ethics consultation – I just wasn't convinced I had done clinical ethics work.

Bourdieu is explicit that when there is some proximity and familiarity between the interviewer and interviewee the possibility of a presumed trust emerges:

> researchers who are socially very close to respondents provide them guarantees against having subjective reasoning reduced to objective causes; of having choices experienced as free turned into objective determinisms uncovered by analysis.[24]

If we're sharing proximity, I'm less likely to imagine a free choice as inevitable because of race, gender, cultural experiences, religious traditions, etc., that I have read about and bring in from outside analysis. Proximity – seeing the person as person and sharing understandings inhibits reading external interpretations into the communication, into the texts and textures of their lives. On the other hand, Bourdieu acknowledges that proximity to the person being questioned puts the questioner at risk and at stake too: "the questioning quite naturally tends to become a double social analysis, one that catches and puts the analysis to the test as much as the person being questioned."[25] If proximity is not acknowledged and accounted for – bracketed – then the work of probing and questioning can redouble back on the interviewer. Proximity puts the questioner into question – including *me* as the consultant/interviewer/questioner. In the *interpretation* of the conversation: the meanings discovered become personally relevant in potentially disruptive ways. As in Bliton's narrative described below, or Schutz's "The Stranger," or as in my MOMS experiences, in the encounter with another person, my own understanding can be thrown into question. The moral engagement can raise questions not only about *how* I understand and *if* I understand – but also about the identity and responsibility of the *I* who is trying to understand.

To be clear, then, when in the role of the interviewer (or the ethics consultant), one acquires multiple responsibilities for what may be relevant, thus requiring awareness of both the social circumstances, commitments, and values of the person being interviewed, as well as one's own social circumstances, commitments, and values. Of course, this awareness helps the interviewer and interviewee negotiate the boundaries between complete overlap where everything is assumed and so cannot be questioned and the complete distance and difference where nothing is assumed and so questions are nonsensical and irrelevant.[26] Not unlike the heightened attention and discipline of Schutz's Stranger, what Bourdieu demands of the interviewer is a kind of "attentiveness to others and a self-abnegation and openness rarely encountered in everyday life."[27] The interviewer, like the Stranger, like the ethics consultant, approaches the other person with a set of ideas about what matters, what is relevant, how to understand the situation at hand, *and yet,* must be willing to suspend and hold those ideas in abeyance to maintain the possibility of understanding and learning from the approached other person. Yet, there are important differences we need to consider between what Schutz describes as the Stranger's experience and the interactions Zaner describes as the ethics consultant's experience, and what Bourdieu expects of the interview in social science research.

Specifically, for Schutz, even when expecting differences between the home community and approached group, between what is known and what is in question, the Stranger is disrupted in the encounter with the other by having to unexpectedly put into question her taken-for-granted ideas and recipes for understanding. The Stranger can't fully know *what* will be disruptive even if she expects and prepares for disruption by the very act of approaching the in-group. Thus, the Stranger's discipline is to anticipate or brace herself for having herself thrown into question by encounters with the Other and is hard won, every time.

Bourdieu's discipline is *expecting* and preparing for one's own disruption *and* being attentive to and aware of and working to minimize the disruption of the others by preparation, education, reflection, and care. However, while aware of the potential disruption to the interviewer, Bourdieu's "Understanding" is most concerned with the potential for the interviewer's disruption of the other – where the interviewer's assumptions and taken for granted recipes can do a kind of violence to and silencing of the other participants. As such, Bourdieu argues that the interviewer is responsible for *beginning* by deliberately shaking off "the inattentive drowsiness induced by the illusion that we've already seen and heard it all,"[28] for beginning from a place of such discipline and care for and attention to the uniqueness of *each* encounter.

The interviewer's preparation includes investigation of these differences and self-reflection that is oriented to and expects disruption by whatever is different and distinct in the interviewee's participation. I had prepared and reviewed both the general frame and my previous experiences, to be open to whatever would reveal itself as important, specifically, to Sally and Theo. I knew I might hear something I'd not heard before, and I knew and was prepared that some families might keep the protective "public face" held up like a mask. I knew the general frame and tried to learn, as Bourdieu insists, by entering "into the distinctive personal history to attempt to gain an understanding – at once unique and general – of each life story."[29] The interviewer, or with Sally and Theo, the ethics consultant, is responsible for being aware of and attentive to the general frames – the backgrounds and contexts that created the possibility for the interview in the first place. Yet those frames cannot be taken for granted as explanatory or presumed to be "common sense," relevant to either the interviewee or to the interviewer. Responsibility for resisting those taken-for-granted understandings falls more heavily on the interviewer than the interviewee and requires deliberate asking about those things which seem most taken-for-granted.

My experience with Sally and Theo in every moment of our conversation, illustrates the weight of that responsibility, inching forwards and away from actually communicating. I was thrown by how unengaged they seemed – dismissive of the questions as "goes without saying" or "mission accomplished!," an avoidance of considering the general questions as relevant to them. Remembering how each question got more difficult to ask, Bourdieu's insistence made sense, that only deep probing of "the tacit presuppositions of common sense can counter the effects of all the representatives of social reality to which both interviewers and interviewees are continually exposed."[30] As a result, the work of the interviewer is thus a unique and deeply unusual type of communication which requires, on the one hand, preparation for and learning about the background frames – the social realities – of the interviewees as well as the interviewer's own social realities. On the other hand, it requires actively suspending, resisting, probing those taken-for-granted, meaning-generating social realities in the attempt to understand what they are and why they matter to the participants in *this* encounter. My general questions inviting Sally and Theo's story of their experiences as well as the more directed inquiry into their understanding of risk and benefit, of God and faith revealed insights and commitments they could share. My questions also exposed the outlines of unspoken values and concerns, meanings that resisted the deep probing I attempted. Theo's question about my role, asked as we wound down the conversation, highlighted that difference and understandings and what is taken for granted. Even after introductions and explanations, they took for granted that they had to answer my questions ... and I took for granted they understood that I was there to help them think through their questions. The disconnect was sharp and difficult to respond to – pointing to another way in which Bourdieu's frame is helpful, as is Mark Bliton's work on the moral elements of practice.[31]

Weaving through all the interviewer's effort and orientation there is, for Bourdieu, a concern and care for the interviewee *in* the encounter, and there is also concern for the interviewer's responsibility to be attuned to the potential disruption of those encounters – for all those involved. Like Zaner's affiliation, Bourdieu's reflexive sociology is a form of and method of attunement – joining with the other in the actual circumstances, seeking to make sense together. Both practices carry a recognition that the disruption can include both the interviewer and interviewee, the consultant and the others with whom he or she engages. The same kind of *bracing for* and willingness to be disrupted emerges in Bliton's account of his clinical ethics experiences and points to the kind of discipline that is required of those who would join in the uncanny with other human beings and their disruption. For Bliton, the potential (or actual) disruption of the clinical ethicist becomes another locus of concern, another thread in the moral tapestry of the clinical encounter that may require attention and care – even within that moment – to mitigate harm to those involved in the consultation – including, explicitly, the consultant. This becomes the third aspect and activity of attunement to consider.

Part of my disruption in the encounter with Sally and Theo occurred after the last conversation with them – after watching the prenatal surgery attempting to repair their son's spina bifida. In a conversation with Sally's father, I experienced a sharp disorientation to my sense of understanding – to what I thought I had learned about Sally from my conversations with her. Sally's dad gave me an unintended reminder of John Hardwig's observation that sometimes we need others to give a more accurate account of our lives – to see things often hidden from the public view.[32]

### Me and the MOMS: ***Thursday***

It was one of the ugliest openings I'd seen.

The hole in the uterus looked like a seared sea urchin, as the surgeon put in stitches and staples in every direction trying to reach homeostasis. When the amniotic fluid came rushing out, an artery in the uterine wall started spurting dark blood, so they had to seal that quickly. The surgeon and team realized the incision was perilously close to the umbilical cord, which had now slithered out over the edge of the uterus.

I was mesmerized by the ropey fragility: whitish blue, iridescent. I'd never seen such a colorful surgery – the dark blood, the blueish sheen of the cord, the white tension spreading across the uterine wall with each contraction. I thought: I prefer less color.

Any time the cord was touched – by surgeon's hand, by the fetus, by the uterine wall – the fetal heart rate would drop. This was the first time I'd heard the cardiologist's voice register anything other than absolute calm. It was such a subtle shift in register that if this had been my first surgery, I wouldn't have noticed it. But she was getting tense. In fact, the whole room was tense.

The carefully rehearsed choreography of repairing the spinal lesion on a fetus still in-utero has always been quiet and calm in the seven surgeries I'd watched so far. The quiet in this one carried foreboding ripples of suppressed panic. And it was intrusive, repeatedly bulldozed flat and to the side by professional discipline. But never quite suppressed.

The incision took longer than usual and was raw, ugly to boot. The surgeons struggled to get the fetus's spine into view so the neurosurgeons could do their work, while the obstetric residents held up the uterus with long strings from the sutures, trying to keep the pressure off the umbilical cord. The fetus and uterus still protested the disruption.

When the cardiologist called out fetal heart rates that were too low, the team paused to let the tiny body recover. Repeatedly, and increasingly often, heads shook, though surgical hands stayed steady. People held their breath while the fetus, through the unstable pressures on the umbilical cord, tried to catch its own.

From the metal stool where I perched, next to the anesthesiologist and nurse anesthetists, looking through the plastic drapes that separated Sally's surgical body from the machinery keeping her breathing safely, I could see. Stitches steadily pulling almost translucent fetal skin closed over fetal spine – I could see the pulling and bunching like fabric caught in a jammed sewing machine. The tissue of fetal skin had torn while final stitches were placed. More heads shaking during the scramble to prepare the artificial skin – AlloDerm – to put under the softly ragged edges – a matrix, a structure where new cells could grow across the gap. The neurosurgeon stepped away while the fellow placed the last stitch and nearly danced their relief – until they caught the eye of their mentor. Calmly seething because the closure had not gone well, knowing he had to call the family with that update, the neurosurgeon headed for the door now that his part of the surgery was over.

I could almost feel my mind dividing itself, trying to listen with one part to the rising tension in the conversation between the neurosurgeons and keeping my gaze and attention on the still gaping abdomen below.

The obstetricians were trying to close out the uterine incision as quickly as possible, while the cardiologist continued to measure out heart rates in a steady voice. They got to the end of the first layer of stitches when the uterus turned white and angry, veins standing out in bas-relief, the just-placed stitches straining against flesh. I bit my gasp behind my teeth before it made noise, and my eyes flicked from one masked face to the next, trying to understand. The surgeon froze, hands ready but not moving. "She's contracting. We need more relaxation. Now." The voice was a near whisper, as if anything louder would undo all their careful work. The nurse anesthetist quietly adjusted dials and the white bulb of the uterus eased its way back toward dusty pink and soft.

The cardiologist reported that the fetal heart rate and cardiac output were going up, her voice still even and calm. The obstetricians went back to placing stitches, blood foaming out where it mixed with saline, injected by the syringe-full to keep the uterus irrigated and replace the lost amniotic fluid. I walked over to stand beside Tori, drawn by her stricken eyes.

"Is everything ok?" My question broke her steel beam gaze toward the still open belly on the table. She spoke softly: "The umbilical cord – you saw it?" I nod.

"The incision was too close to the cord – makes it hard to work without squeezing the cord – and of course, that's the source of blood and oxygen for the fetus. That's what caused all the fetal distress – the dips in heart rate and output. But this is also how we lost the baby in surgery before: the cord got looped in one of the stitches during closure. The uterus started contracting and they had to open everything back up again – fast. They almost lost the mom, too, that time."

She shook her head out of the memory and patted my hand, gripping the elbow closest to her as I kept my body in tight. She nodded again toward the now nearly closed skin: "Almost done. Now we've got to keep that baby in that belly a couple of weeks. Then we'll see what happens."

I nodded, hearing her but not sure if I understood what I'd seen, what was happening next. How could I make sense of the near tragedy, in that operating room? After seeing in technicolor the very thing I'd been unable to get Sally and Theo to consider, how could I go forward in the morass of horror and wonder and clinical calm, into their uncertain futures, to talk with them, or those taking care of them? I stood very still and quiet.

### Mark J. Bliton: Self-Reflexivity and the Trembling of Attunement

As I tried to make sense of this encounter – at the time and even now – I turned to my preparation and to previous experience, even if that experience was not my own. In his 2008 essay, "Maternal Fetal Surgery and the Profoundest Question in Ethics"[33] Mark Bliton explores the experience of attunement – of joining with another in their questions and uncertainty and unknowing – in their disruption and need to know. This becomes our need to know, as ethics consultants, and our responsibility for attending to and responding to what is most relevant to those with whom we are engaged. Bliton invites recognition of that responsibility even when doing so creates disruption and risks to ourselves.

Written for a collection gathered and edited by two of Zaner's and Bliton's former students and colleagues, Denise Dudzinski and Paul Ford, "The Profoundest Question" tells the story of an old case – one that "haunts," per the book's theme. In Bliton's account, he retells his engagement with questions about *his* experience and *his* responsibilities, which emerged in the consultation. In this reflection, re-remembered several times per his own telling, Bliton gives the narrative of a clinical ethics consultation regarding prenatal surgery for spina bifida, which ended with a fetal demise. Bliton describes his "uncanny" encounter with the patient and patient's mother, after the failed surgery, and being shown the lovingly swaddled body of the dead fetus.

Bliton's reflection on the narrative of his experience, reveals this as a disruptive encounter with the uncanny – when the individual is "seized by what is primordially strange"[34] – that occurred from within his role as an ethics consultant. He reflects that the act of self-reflection into "our own sense of values inherent in the performance and activities of ethics consultation"[35] is not an easy one (nor, as Frolic would amplify, a profoundly common one). Bliton suggests that as ethics consultants, when confronted by the intimate experiences of illness, injury, disability, and dying, that challenge the *basis* for our values, we prefer to move right along and hold fast to the taken-for-granted values that generally guide our work. In encounters with the uncanny, "ethics consultants may be confronted with implications or insights into their own understandings – or misunderstandings – about those beliefs and values most cherished to themselves, and maybe to others."[36]

Or, as has been raised by Ofstad and Frolic, Wolff, and Zaner, Bliton makes explicit that in ethics consultation, there is an inherent, baked-in, unavoidable moral experience of "the individual's discovery of his/her humanity – and the fact that he or she lacks important and real knowledge about what that means."[37] Further, and perhaps most crucially, this discovery and its meaning occur in relationships and situations and even in the body into which one is thrown, unchosen.

### Unspeakable Responsibility

Bliton notes, then, that "one crucial sense of 'moral' … is encountered precisely in the dramatic shift of attention by a 'self' to the latent vulnerability of embodiment, accident, and chance shared with other person and evoked in the experiences of the threatened, impaired, or dying other."[38] The moral element of the encounter is the disruption, the recognition, the process of becoming receptive to and aware of what is shared with the other. The ethics consultant's moral responsibility emerges in the recognition of, attention to, and responsiveness to that encountered disruption when they face the question of how to go forward in that relationship, to help, to learn without causing harm that is apparent from within that shared encounter.

In doing clinical ethics work, we find a demand and responsibility to be constantly vigilant to our uncanny encounters – and resist the urge to move right along, even with all the justifications we generate to allow us to skate over the shaky parts. But if we don't resist, we can create harm to the person or people who are caught in their unchosen, often-uncanny experiences. We can create harm on a professional level – to clinical ethics practice and integrity – because we may miss something crucial, and so not fulfill our role responsibility,[39] and not fulfill our professional responsibility for ongoing learning. And we may cause deep damage to ourselves – *as humans* who happen to be clinical ethics consultants. Unprocessed moral disruption and the disequilibrium that follows can create blinders and toughen scars that inhibit our moral engagements and interactions beyond our work: soul damage and moral injury are not to be taken lightly.

Thus, Bliton drills down to an often overlooked (perhaps deliberately avoided?) core question about one's responsibility as an ethics consultant, *for the consultant* themself and in relationship with others: "Is it more harmful or beneficial to identify and articulate crucial factors that remain unspoken, possibility unacknowledged, and perhaps unimagined?"[40] How is one to go forward, probe further in the face of disruption and distress, or conversely, how does one hold back when the disruption that threatens to overwhelm also may highlight what is most important? Bliton breaks this conundrum down further into two points with relevance to the process and experience of attunement.

First, Bliton emphasizes that while preparation and methodology may identify needed areas for inquiry and suggest approaches *to* the questions, it is only *in* the encounter that one can discover the *actual* questions-at-hand – and whether or even how to probe them. The attunement – being ac-climated to or aware of such potential disruptions is necessary, foremost because, as Bliton notes, people may not want to (or may not be able to) "examine themselves in that focus of tormented choices, despairing commitments, and furtive allegiances in their own lives."[41] For example, in the MOMS interview with Sally and Theo, the question of faith as guidance for decision-making emerged as more relevant to one partner than the other – but the other partner did not take the invi-tation to probe or give a different account of the faith narrative offered by their spouse. Is pursuing such questions helpful? Harmful? What is the responsibility if there are clear indicators that one's interlocuter does not want to pursue the questions? In ethics consultation – even or especially for an experimental procedure like prenatal surgery for spina bifida – the ethics consultant is in rela-tionship and communication with someone in a deeply vulnerable position and so is obligated to a deep responsibility for non-harm or, now taking Bourdieu to heart, responsibility for avoiding violence. The ethics consultant must be both prepared to ask and attuned to their responsibility for the whether and how of asking – even to being prepared for not-asking.

### What, Then, Is Left?

The whether-and-how to ask raises another question, however, and leads to the second point of Bliton's concern: "If ethics consultants shy away from and do not articulate and rigorously exam-ine such influential dispositions, values, and beliefs, then what is left of ethics?"[42] In talking with Sally and Theo, I fully faced the wrenching difficulty of Bliton's question. I tried various types of indirection and invitation and I was reflexively aware of the limits of asking further. I felt the lay-ers and boundaries through which I could not press without asserting a power and authority not authorized simply by my being in that role: to help, to understand, to learn, to make space for them to speak what they needed. While committed to learning and helping in the MOMS interview with Sally and Theo, part of what I discovered in the attunement was the limits of my commitments – and the difficult-to-articulate but very real sense of danger to those I was trying to help. How could I engage in the ethical concerns discovered and emerging in these moments? How could I respond to the limits of their needs and experiences yet not get so caught by their overwhelm that I lost the ability or will to pursue, from my experiences and within my commitments, what I understood as important in this type of "ethics" discussion.

The challenging experiences captured in the MOMS self-reflections above mirror the experi-ence in Bliton's account: wondering, as the ethics consultant, if I dared to pursue the questions and themes that seemed to generate resistance, that seemed to indicate "here there be monsters," where we find the sticking points. How could I proceed when those who are opening themselves to conversation with me are showing me their limits? In the conversations, the deliberate pursuit of some of my questions, and engagement with Sally and Theo, I discovered a particular kind of limit, a point at which the uncanny, the mystery, the thrown-ness of their surrender would not be contained or caught by further probing. In the process of attunement, I recognized that we had reached a point of understanding, had done so together, and, perhaps most crucially, had recognized a limit of understanding that demanded restraint in my activities as a clinical ethics consultant or researcher.

I do not take from Bliton's reflection that the ethics consultant is the arbiter and decider of what is ethically relevant and hence must be addressed and to what level of fullness or completion in any consultation. Rather, in his question there lies the deep concern for ethics as a practice of moral inquiry, not a set of pre-established questions or fully anticipated answers.

The ethics consultant has to prepare, like Bourdieu, and to go in with some idea of what is at stake – what might need to be addressed or probed. And the ethics consultant is responsible for attention and discovery and response if another concern is *actually* at stake and needs to be addressed. Similarly, the ethics consultant must be attuned to the limits that become evident and be prepared to stop before causing harm. But none of this is presupposed or prefigured, which is the great scandal of *clinical* ethics in comparison to applied ethics or process ethics or even bioethics broadly understood. In clinical ethics, the work is *always* individual and personal, it is always attention, self-reflection and attunement that lead to decisions – to thought, judgment, actions of the ethics consultant in the moment of consultation. The ethics consultant may not bear the final responsibility for what happens or the outcome, but they do bear the responsibility for their own comportment, action, reflection in each encounter. And to bear that responsibility with integrity means carrying the full acknowledgment of their own limitations, biases, particularities – *humanness* that may be influential beyond their intentions. It means resisting the shelter and escape of claims that the individual ethics consultant is not responsible because they are using legal frames, or standardized practices and guidelines. They are still deciding which elements make it fitting, and that is the weight and responsibility on the clinical ethics consultant. So, the ethics consultant must own their judgments and assessments as well as their particular skills – and limitations – which means the consultant and their practice must always be available for inquiry and investigation too.

The ethics consultant is responsible for following the "discipline of the problem" – identifying, attuning, and responding to the issues and concerns that reveal themselves in the context – including ones that the ethics consultant may carry into the situations and conversations – intentionally or not. Rather than remaining wedded to external or pre-existing frames of what is at stake and what really matters, the ethics consultant must carry a relentless inquiry: they must resist the formalities and assumptions that can mask the unfolding and discovery of each consultation encounter. Enacting such responsibility requires, in fact, an element of trust in oneself, as well as trust in those with whom one is engaged: living into an assumption that by participating, all are working toward mutual understanding, and doing so carefully – as in, doing so with extra-ordinary care, in an extra-ordinary discourse.

## Me and the MOMS: ***Thursday Afternoon***

People were leaving the operating room. I followed along, not knowing what else to do or where else to go. Everyone around me moved with purpose and toward their next task. Tori saw my hesitation and waved me forward until I was walking behind her and the transport nurse pushing the gurney. Next to him, Sally's nurse shepherded the wheeled IV pole, draped with cords and lines still attached to Sally's arms.

The procession felt solemn: I actively erased thoughts of "funereal" as they intruded. I didn't know if the quiet was normal – out of respect to the pregnant woman still groggy from anesthesia? Or if it was in response to the near catastrophes of the surgery today? I'd never been a part of this part – every time we'd watched a surgery before, Mark and I left the operating room, changed out of and returned our borrowed scrubs, and walked slowly back to the conference room in the Center for Clinical and Research Ethics, reflecting on the experience. This time, I was still *in* the experience.

We crossed into the Labor and Delivery unit, with cheerful pastel walls. Tori walked ahead of me through the door of Sally's room into a bustle of activity and conversation. Tori immediately went toward the bed to help the L&D nurse get Sally settled and connect the dangling IVs to the right monitors and plugs on the wall.

I melted myself into the wall by the door, listening to snatches of conversation. The mothers fussed over Sally, and Tori spoke with Theo about the surgery and what the neurosurgeon had shared about needing to use the AlloDerm. I wondered if that was all they'd shared – if the terrible opening and bone white contractions and dipping fetal heartrate were held back. I guessed so, but still wondered, and didn't know who or how – or whether to ask in a way that wouldn't sound accusatory, as if I thought I knew that they should be. Tori was busy showing Theo and Sally pictures of the baby's spine and everyone commented on how big the lesion was, on how glad they were for the prenatal surgery – to close that giant hole before it caused damage.

Sally's dad sidled over during this phase and whispered, "I don't really want to see. I'm just glad *my* baby is back up here and safe." I smiled at him. His obvious sense of displacement created an odd mirror to mine. He continued chatting while we both watched the activity and conversation around Sally and Theo. "So, what does the MTS on your badge mean?" he asked.

I smiled again. Most people don't know about the abbreviation for Masters of Theological Studies. When I explained about my degree from the Divinity School and my current doctoral studies in religion and ethics, he opened up.

"That's really neat! Theo and his family are Catholic – very Catholic. We're Episcopalian – Catholic Lite." He chuckled and continued. "When the kids first got the diagnosis, we wondered if they would think about abortion. I wondered if it would be better than bringing a child into the world with all this suffering from birth."

I nodded, encouragingly, actively wondering how this went in their family dynamics. "I asked Sally too, just me and her one day, if she'd thought about it. She said she had, but she didn't want to be selfish, to put her worries above the baby's needs. Plus," he grimaced, "Theo would have hit the roof if she'd really considered it. They're *really* Catholic."

I looked at him, trying to process these new insights as quickly as I could, trying to figure out how to respond. I looked instead at his daughter, the groggy woman on the bed, her hand fluttering toward the solid form of her husband. She looked so different from the woman I'd sat across the conference room table from 48 hours ago, and for just a moment, I saw her through her dad's experience: large and containing multitudes, struggling to figure out what was right for her and for her family. I squirmed inside, shifted my weight on my feet as I realized she no longer fit into the defined judgments I'd formed through our interactions: maybe I hadn't understood her nearly as much as I imagined.

Sally's dad sighed, "You know, we are so proud of her for taking on this burden – not that this child is a burden! He's a blessing! But taking on all this extra responsibility, rather than the easy way out. I mean, I know a lot of women get abortions."

I resisted the urge to educate him on the fallacy of a second trimester abortion as an "easy way out" and so took a breath before responding. "It's a tough choice for many women, but the families we see in the MOMS trial have already decided against abortion, mostly." He smiled and nodded. Was that satisfaction at being part of a small group? Hard to tell. I continued.

"Even with the extra responsibility and challenges, these families are going to take care of their children in the best ways they can. These kids often do well no matter which surgery they get, because their parents are so willing to do whatever it takes for them."

He smiled again, nodding decisively. "Well, little Theo has a family that will do that, that's for sure."

He said a quick thanks and walked over toward his daughter and wife, as Tori was saying her goodbyes. I added mine, with thanks and well wishes for Sally and Baby Theo.

Tori and I closed the door on our way out.

### The Conditions for Extra-Ordinary Discourse

Part of what resonates between Bourdieu and clinical ethics work is Bourdieu's articulation of the research relationship and the responsibilities of the interviewer (to the interviewee, as well as to the interview itself) as creating "an absolutely exceptional situation for communication."[43] Unlike everyday speech or interactions, where the taken-for-granted social roles and expectations, as well as limitations of time and access, shape and constrain what can be said or what is known, the interview process becomes an opportunity for "opening up alternatives which prompt or authorize the articulation of worries, needs, or wishes, discovered through this very articulation."[44] In the space created by and rigorously maintained by the interviewer's discipline, the interviewee – the person with the most at stake in the communication – can take advantage of the "conditions for an extraordinary discourse, which might never have been spoken, but was already there, merely waiting for the conditions of its authorization."[45] The interviewer's attention, knowledge, deep engagement with the individual present in the particular moments of the encounter is part of a discipline offering a way to see, to engage with the other person and what matters *as they present themselves in the encounter,* rather than seeing an individual as a type, or relying on our social cues and taken-for-granted recipes for making sense of their experience and understanding.

For Bourdieu, the interview or conversation "can be considered as a sort of *spiritual exercise* that, through forgetfulness of self, aim(ed) at a true *conversion* of *the way we look* at other people in the ordinary circumstances of life."[46] Not unlike how Kurt Wolff describes surrender-and-catch as an experience of cognitive love,[47] Bourdieu describes his work as an orientation or a becoming as much as a rigorous method, where "the welcoming disposition, which leads one to make the respondent's problems one's own, the capacity to take that person just as they are in their distinctive necessity, is a sort of intellectual love."[48] In the movement between the unique and the general, the discovered amid the presumed, the transcendent irrupting into the mundane, the other person draws one's complete attention, such that received notions and recipes for understanding shift out of focus and the interviewer, like Wolff's investigator, surrenders to their unknowing and their trying to understand.

In a similar vein, as in these descriptions about interviews and investigation, in clinical ethics work, the practices include learning how to probe and consider and reflect on both the topic and concern at hand and one's own commitments and values and taken for granted recipes. These practice elements can be (and, indeed, must be) developed and cultivated as pre-requisites for asking others to do so and inviting such extra-ordinary communication. Further, and more challenging, the interviewer and the ethics consultant must continue such learning – and be attentive to the limits of their preparation, understanding, and communication *in the midst of* such conversations. As Bourdieu notes, the interviewer (as with the ethics consultant) is responsible for constructing discourses and investigations "scientifically, in such a way that it yields the elements necessary for its own explanation."[49] The interviewer/ethics consultant has a responsibility for creating the conditions for and possibility of collaboratively constructing meaning within the conversation, for and with the other with whom they are engaged in such extra-ordinary discourse.

The practice of careful attunement requires being able to say what one is thinking, to reveal one's self-reflections, to communicate the catch/understanding that follows the surrender-to/questioning in clinical ethics and research work. As with Wolff's surrender-and-catch, the responsibility in clinical ethics consultation continues beyond the attunement and the encounter: the consultant finds herself responsible for communicating, for sharing the catch with others – and doing so faithfully, fairly, as accurately as possible, for the possibility of learning even after the encounter. Especially when that catch is a story, a lesson, an understanding gleaned from the moral life of those in difficult circumstances, accessed by attunement and elicited through affiliation.

*Afterwards/After Words*

It felt rehearsed, like a performance piece. Which feels like a pot-and-kettle judgment since I had actually rehearsed and memorized the questions I might need to ask. Perhaps she practiced and memorized the answers she might have to give. But our rehearsals were at cross purposes and I could feel it in the tensions of the conversation.

I aimed my rehearsals to open the conversation wherever it needed to go. But I also had visions, imaginings, preconceived assumptions about what that direction might look like. I discovered how strongly I held those and took them for granted only when they came up hard against Sally's rehearsed performance.

Her practice was directed toward getting into the trial – she said what she knew to say. She had thought about the issues and concerns that I had learned needed to be considered: the risks, the research aspect, the randomization. It was obvious she'd done her homework and educated herself about all the practicalities. But the conversation remained closed, despite all the appearances of and opportunities for openness. Sally gave a series of reports, rather than a personal account: studied lines, rather than reflective responses. As I wrote in my journal at the time – *my* report, as it were, for Mark to review with me after his return to town:

> *Theo had more affect than Sally did, which made him seem more open and engaged, as if he were following the questions and the conversation. The sense from Sally was tense, but not in the typically fragile way – it was more a numbness that I've seen a few times before – as if she just wanted it to be over. And these are not impressions I articulated to myself in the conversation, but in reflecting on it afterwards.*

And yet, even beyond my insights and assessments, the meanings I did glean and learn from Sally, she still exceeded the encounter and my understanding. As my conversation with Sally's dad reminded me, there is always more than is shared, is visible, than can be understood by the ethics consultant – and perhaps by the very people with whom she endeavors to help. "Sally" and "Theo" – in all their iterations and variations that I've met over the years – are EveryPatient and EveryFamily. They are also their own unique selves – demanding both preparation and experience along with my utter naiveté and openness and curiosity about their lives, their experiences, and their concerns. And I am both EveryEthicsConsultant – and my own radically unique self – which means in my professional role, I myself must be subject to the same preparation and experience, curiosity and openness about my experiences, my concerns, my practice. I am not exempt from the risk and opportunity, the vulnerability that such extraordinary discourse – attunement – prompts and requires.

## Notes

1  The Management of Myelomeningocele Study (MOMS trial) was a randomized controlled clinical trial evaluating the outcomes of open-uterine prenatal surgery to repair spina bifida versus post-natal standard of care. Adzick, N. Scott, Elizabeth A. Thom, Catherine Y. Spong, John W. Brock III, Pamela K. Burrows, Mark P. Johnson, Lori J. Howell, et al. (2011). A randomized trial of prenatal versus postnatal repair of myelomeningocele. *New England Journal of Medicine* 364 (11):993–1004; Bartlett, Virginia L. and Bliton, Mark J. (2020). Retrieving the moral in the ethics of maternal-fetal surgery. *Cambridge Quarterly of Healthcare Ethics* 29 (3):480–493.

2  Zaner, Richard M. (2015). *A Critical Examination of Ethics in Health Care and Biomedical Research: Voices and Visions*. Springer. pp. 143–144 (hereafter VAV).

3  Zaner. *VAV*, 145.

4  In *Phenomenology and the Clinical Event*, Zaner describes "fertilizing one's imagination" with previous experiences and free-phantasy variation" – i.e., imaginatively varying the features of a presented situation

to make clear which features are constant and essential. See Zaner, Richard M. (1994). Phenomenology and the Clinical Event. In M. Daniel and Lester E. Embree (eds.), *Phenomenology and the Cultural Disciplines*. Boston: Kluwer Academic Publishers. pp. 39–66 (hereafter PCE).

5  *Ibid.* 40.
6  Zaner, PCE, fn 3.
7  Bourdieu, Pierre J. (1999). Understanding. In Pierre Bourdieu (ed.), *The Weight of the World: Social Suffering in Contemporary Society*. Cambridge, UK: Polity Press. pp. 607–626.
8  Bliton Mark J. (2008). Maternal-Fetal Surgery and the 'Profoundest Question in Ethics.' In: Paul J. Ford and Denise M. Dudzinski (eds.), *Complex Ethics Consultations: Cases That Haunt Us*. Cambridge, UK: Cambridge University Press. pp. 36–42.
9  Zaner, PCE, 40.
10 Zaner, PCE, 39–40.
11 *Ibid.* 40.
12 *Ibid.*
13 Zaner, R.M. (2010). On the Telling of Stories. In Osborne P. Wiggins and Annette Allen (eds.), *Ethics and Histories in Clinical Medicine: Essays in Honor of Richard M. Zaner*. Springer. p. 202 (hereafter TOS).
14 *Ibid.* 203.
15 Zaner, PCE, 47.
16 Zaner, PCE, 49–52, 53–61.
17 *Ibid.* 59.
18 *Ibid.* 50.
19 Bourdieu, "Understanding" 608.
20 *Ibid.* 608.
21 *Ibid.* 609.
22 *Ibid.* 609.
23 Bishop, Jeffrey P. (2018). Doing Well or Doing Good in Ethics Consultation. In Stuart G. Finder and Mark J. Bliton (eds.), *Peer Review, Peer Education, and Modeling in the Practice of Clinical Ethics Consultation: The Zadeh Project*. Cham, Switzerland: Springer Verlag. pp. 179–192.
24 Bourdieu, "Understanding," 610.
25 *Ibid.* 611.
26 *Ibid.* 612.
27 *Ibid.*
28 *Ibid.* 614.
29 *Ibid.*
30 *Ibid.* 620.
31 Bliton Mark J. (2008). Maternal-Fetal Surgery and the 'Profoundest Question in Ethics.' In Paul J. Ford and Denise M. Dudzinski (eds.), *Complex Ethics Consultations: Cases That Haunt Us*. Cambridge, UK: Cambridge University Press. pp. 36–42.
32 Hardwig, J. (1997). Autobiography, Biography, and Narrative Ethics. In H. Lindeman (ed.), *Stories and Their Limits: Narrative Approaches to Bioethics*. New York, NY: Routledge. pp. 50–64.
33 Bliton, "Profoundest Question," 36–42.
34 Natanson, Maurice (1998). *The Erotic Bird: Phenomenology in Literature*. Princeton, NJ: Princeton University Press. pp. 54, 133.
35 Bliton, "Profoundest Question," 38.
36 *Ibid.* 39.
37 *Ibid.*
38 *Ibid.*
39 Finder, S. G. and Bliton, M. J. (2001). Activities, not rules: The need for responsive practice (on the way toward responsibility). *American Journal of Bioethics* 1 (4):52–54.
40 Bliton, "Profoundest Question," 40.
41 *Ibid.* 40.
42 Bliton, "Profoundest Question," 40.
43 Bourdieu, "Understanding," p. 614.
44 *Ibid.*
45 *Ibid.*
46 *Ibid.*

47 Wolff, Kurt H. (1976). Surrender and Catch: Experience and Inquiry Today. In *Boston Studies in the Philosophy and History of Science*, vol. 51. Dordrecht: Springer.
48 Bourdieu, "Understanding," p. 614.
49 *Ibid.* 611.

## Bibliography

Adzick, N. Scott, Thom, Elizabeth A., Spong, Catherine Y., Brock, John W. III, Burrows, Pamela K., Johnson, Mark P., and Howell, Lori J., et al. (2011). A randomized trial of prenatal versus postnatal repair of myelomeningocele. *New England Journal of Medicine* 364 (11): 993–1004.
Bartlett, Virginia L. and Bliton, Mark J. (2020). Retrieving the moral in the ethics of maternal-fetal surgery. *Cambridge Quarterly of Healthcare Ethics* 29 (3):480–493.
Bishop, Jeffrey P. (2018). Doing Well or Doing Good in Ethics Consultation. In Stuart G. Finder and Mark J. Bliton (eds.), *Peer Review, Peer Education, and Modeling in the Practice of Clinical Ethics Consultation: The Zadeh Project*. Cham, Switzerland: Cham, Switzerland: Springer Verlag. pp. 179–192.
Bliton, Mark J. (2008). Maternal-Fetal Surgery and the 'Profoundest Question in Ethics'. In Paul J. Ford and Denise M. Dudzinski (eds.), *Complex Ethics Consultations: Cases That Haunt Us*. Cambridge, UK: Cambridge University Press. pp. 36–42.
Bourdieu, P.J. (1999). Understanding. In Pierre Bourdieu (ed.), *The Weight of the World: Social Suffering in Contemporary Society*. Cambridge, UK: Polity Press. pp. 607–626.
Finder, S. G. and Bliton, M. J. (2001). Activities, not rules: The need for responsive practice (on the way toward responsibility). *American Journal of Bioethics* 1 (4): 52–54.
Hardwig, J. (1997). Autobiography, Biography, and Narrative Ethics. In H. Lindeman (ed.), *Stories and Their Limits: Narrative Approaches to Bioethics*. New York, NY: Routledge. pp. 50–64.
Natanson, Maurice (1998). *The Erotic Bird: Phenomenology in Literature*. Princeton, NJ: Princeton University Press.
Wolff, Kurt H. (1976). Surrender and Catch: Experience and Inquiry Today. In *Boston Studies in the Philosophy and History of Science*, vol. 51. Dordrecht: Springer.
Zaner, Richard M. (1994). Phenomenology and the Clinical Event. In M. Daniel and Lester E. Embree (eds.), *Phenomenology and the Cultural Disciplines*. Boston, MA: Kluwer Academic Publishers. pp. 39–66.
Zaner, R.M. (2010). On the Telling of Stories. In Osborne P. Wiggins and Annette Allen (eds.), Ethics and Histories in Clinical Medicine: Essays in Honor of Richard M. Zaner. Cham, Switzerland: Springer.
Zaner, Richard M. (2015). *A Critical Examination of Ethics in Health Care and Biomedical Research: Voices and Visions*. Cham, Switzerland: Springer. pp. 143–144.

# Interlude II: Methods for Learning with Others

## Vulnerability and Sharing Stories

### From Attunement to Vulnerability

Responsible clinical ethics work both invites and requires engagement with others in the field to critically interrogate and learn about what all matters for each consultant. Frolic's self-reflection, Ofstad's moral development, Zaner's attunement, Bourdieu's sociological eye, and Bliton's affiliation are lenses that bring focus to the ethics consultant's deeply intentional, and even personal, involvement in whatever situation prompts the conversation with a patient or family or clinician. The ethics consultant's self-understanding may be at stake in the questions at hand in a consultation (and often long "after" it ends[1]), and so they carry an interwoven responsibility and vulnerability in the encounter. It is these personal and the interpersonal interactions that allow for meanings and understandings to develop and be communicated – and then be considered and become the basis for current and future activities and choices.

While these implications might seem so evident as to be unnecessary to mention, how they occur, and the ways practical meanings develop, may be so deeply embedded in the practice of clinical ethics consultation as to be obscured, even for those whose practice is at stake. As philosopher and writer Robert M. Pirsig notes, "it occurred to me that there *is* no manual that deals with the *real* business ... the most important aspect of all. Caring about what you're doing is considered either unimportant or taken for granted."[2] Pirsig voiced his concerns through the lens of motorcycle maintenance, but his observations hold true for paying attention to any activities or experiences about which we care – including, in this context, our personal experiences as ethics consultants. He cautions, "When you want to hurry something, that means you no longer care about it and want to get on to other things. I just want to get at it slowly, but carefully and thoroughly."[3] Being careful and thorough, sharing our practice, especially by writing and giving thick descriptions and detailed accounts of that practice, gives us the opportunity to get at it slowly, carefully, thoroughly, not rushing ahead for the object lesson or takeaway point. Doing so, however, brings a peculiar level of exposure to things that matter to us in the doing. Sharing our stories, in contrast to constructing our conventional cases, illuminates a connection between the work we do and the vulnerability we encounter while doing it.

The vulnerability that comes with responsibility, especially the practices of being attuned to and affiliated with the other people in their crisis, is so rarely discussed in the field of clinical ethics consultation that when consultants *do* share stories of their experiences, they stand out and demand attention. Instead, we read or hear, "This is a classic case of conflict between autonomy and beneficence," or "The process lacked ..." or "The consultant did *x* instead of *y*." Or, the clinical ethics encounters are framed as anonymized examples of *kinds* of ethical issues or disease or demographic types: "For end-of-life cases we ..." or "This is about patients with dementia ..." Even those brazen enough to try sharing their stories face the challenge of being misunderstood as

DOI: 10.4324/9781003354864-9

offering them as fodder for evaluation of the ethicality of a case or outcome, whether the proce-dural conventionalism of one's consultation "fit" the case. Yet clinical stories are as different from clinical cases as peer learning or education is different from peer review.

### *Learning about Our Own Practice Requires Help from Others*

The elements of practice I discussed in Part II, through both the stories of clinical ethics experi-ences and drawing from Frolic, Ofstad, Bourdieu, Zaner, and Bliton, are illustrations of moments in the actual *doing* of clinical ethics – in individual practice and as practitioners in a field that claims, like a profession, to learn together. The type of self-reflection and self-education or moral develop-ment identified by Frolic and Ofstad demands engagement with others who are willing to join in the uncertainty and vulnerability. To listen and tell with an openness to discovering meaning and trying to make sense of these encounters, rather than retreating to the conventions of a kind of distanced comfort, one that already presumes that there is a type of a certainty available in such crises. That distancing can just a readily end up being reductive and misplaced, almost intentionally avoid-ing the discomfort and uncertainties. In contrast, attunement and affiliation realize the existential and interpersonal: the nitty-gritty, mundane, face-to-face interactions. There are also moments of transcendence, large and small, in these mundane human experiences: the connections that exceed and escape the rationalities and analytic structures we use to contain the crisis of uncertainty, the vulnerability generated by illness and injury, and the commitments to caring for other humans.

Self-reflection or self-education, as well as attunement and affiliation, are not always recognized as elements of practice because they can so easily get subsumed under the procedural or bureau-cratic concerns, by conceptual analyses that disfavor the normative messiness of the personal and interpersonal. As a result, even when not present, not to mention when inactive, self-reflection and self-education are assumed to be part of practice, primarily due to the presumed prestige associated with the vocabularies of "ethics." Hence, they are easily overlooked, and yet remain constituent elements of method in clinical ethics work that help us take seriously our engagement, just as the elements of disruption, attention, and surrender-and-catch which Part I explored. In this context, sharing stories of actual ethics encounters is not an easy or comfortable experience, whether you are the one sharing these stories, or the one encountering them as a reader. It very well may be that the revelation of differences, along with actions and ideas which seem strange in each other's practice is unnerving at a time when, in our field, the commitment of professionalization as stand-ardization is strong. Thus, learning how to share our stories and how to engage with the stories other people share becomes a part of practice that also needs attention, modeling, and discussion.

### Engaging with *the Zadeh Project*: Peer Review as Peer Learning

The most helpful example of this kind of sharing and meaning-making about clinical ethics con-sultation is a recent work, a collaborative project edited by Stuart G. Finder and Mark J. Bliton. Published in 2018, *Peer Review, Peer Education, and Modeling in the Practice of Clinical Ethics Consultation: The Zadeh Project* addresses the continually challenging question of how ethics consultants can learn from each other.[4] Over the course of ten years, Finder and Bliton shared a long-form clinical case narrative that emerged from one of Finder's consultation experiences – "the Zadeh Scenario" – with peers across the US and internationally, seeking feedback and insights from others, with the narrative as a shared starting point and touchstone.[5] The project became an iterative, layered example of the possibilities – and pitfalls – of peer learning in clinical ethics consultation.

The Zadeh Scenario underwent three rounds of review and commentary.[6] The first reviewers focused on the narrative itself and what it revealed or raised regarding clinical ethics consultation.

The second group of reviewers offered commentary on the narrative and on the first-round reviews, specifically considering method or methodology in practice. The third round of reviewers commented on the scenario as well as the previous two rounds, focusing on peer review and peer learning as a process. After unfolding through several conference panels at the International Conference on Clinical Ethics Consultation, Bliton and Finder edited the texts into a rich and fascinating book, published under Springer's open-access model, to be available to all who might be interested in engaging such questions.

*The Zadeh Project* stands out as a document and resource in both what it reveals about practice (through the Scenario and the commentaries) and what it reveals about the challenges and rewards of attempting to learn with and through engagement with others in the field. As an orientation and approach to practice, as a practice of peer learning, and as a thoughtfully constructed book, *the Zadeh Project* elicits engagement from peers – with explicit acknowledgment of the differences in practice and orientation – for the benefit of the field as a whole. With the widely different perspectives of the contributors, *The Zadeh Project* illustrates the kind of learning about practice that Ofstad described as interpersonal, mutual growth, or that Frolic – in earlier work – articulated as self-reflection about one's embodied, personal practice. Peer learning, then, *can* be an experience of invitation and attunement, of "listening-and-telling" of the kind described by Zaner, and by Finder and Bliton.[7] Like Bourdieu's interviewer with the reflective reflexivity of the sociological eye, a reader or reviewer with enough background and affiliation can engage another's clinical ethics story, such that not everything is in question because of what is shared (enough) as participants in the field of clinical ethics, *and yet* the reader/reviewer can have enough recognition of their own historicity and peculiar particularity (à la Wolff) to where not everything is assumed to be known and understood. Peer learning, through stories of the kind modeled in *the Zadeh Project*, is an opportunity to question together what it is we do and why, to reassess, to reconsider in the multitude of our individual and institutional contexts, what might be fitting and why as part of developing practice.[8]

### *Interpersonal and Individual Vulnerability: Reflections on the Zadeh Project and Sharing Stories with Strangers*

*The Zadeh Project* engages the kinds of mutual self-reflection and self-education that become a caring, attuned kind of practice, in affiliation with others in the field. *The Zadeh Project* – as an endeavor and a publication – illustrates and embodies a kind of attunement and trust required to tell stories, to share our experiences of clinical encounters that are unabashedly about *us as clinical ethics consultants*. It also illustrates some of the disconnects in that process of sharing stories. Even among well-intentioned and thoughtful peers, we all have a hard time getting deep into our own commitments, in order to move beyond those, and possibly hear and understand what our peers are actually saying. The thorough engagement in *the Zadeh Project*, the care and attention with which participants engaged the experiential narrative and the various questions about method, evaluation, and peer learning identifies opportunities and even requirements for ongoing engagement as a field. Specifically, two themes emerged from the collection that were absolutely stunning, and together, point to the final two elements of responsibility in *Sharing Stories with Strangers*.

First, the repeated acknowledgement, even praise, for the vulnerability Finder revealed and courage required for him to share his own experience so thoroughly and openly was remarkable: "generously revealed"[9] "rich narrative generously shared"[10] and "outstanding, thoughtful, self-critical narrative"[11] and "makes himself vulnerable in this new mechanism for peer review."[12] **The Zadeh Project reveals the recognition, perhaps unwelcome, that articulating one's practice and demonstrating one's commitments is now a radical and rare activity in our field.** Recognizing that it is now a rare and radical act to talk explicitly about what we actually do in daily practice is deeply troubling. Why is being open about one's own uncertainty and experience of vulnerability is seen as awe-inspiring and unique? Especially for a field of practitioners who purport to engage in others' uncertainty and vulnerability in their day-to-day work? Why is there a deep disconnect between the vulnerability of patients, families, and clinical colleagues and our own vulnerability, such that describing and engaging and reflecting on the former is taken for granted as foundational to the work, while describing and engaging the latter is strange enough to be noteworthy, even praiseworthy?

*The Zadeh Project* illustrates the vulnerability we reveal when we talk explicitly about our own practice – and our discomfort with sharing those embodied, particular, historical experiences. *The Zadeh Project* also reveals the difficulty we have in learning from our own and each other's experiences. We get caught by and reveal our own commitments and values which then require further attention and self-reflection, and like the taken-for-granted recipes from the Stranger's home community, may not be adequate or fitting for the situations in which we find ourselves. Which leads to the second theme that emerges from *the Zadeh Project*, especially considering the elements of practice outlined in Part II: *that responsible clinical ethics consultation requires grappling with vulnerability – and that means doing so through telling our own stories.*

Sharing stories about ourselves is more than just presenting consults in the form of a publishing a case report or giving an institutional presentation, or even swapping "war stories" in the coffee bar at a professional conference. As an intentional practice, sharing stories can be a rigorous and thorough means of learning together – which means it is also a risky one. For individuals, sharing stories about our actual practice is risky because it draws explicit attention to the double vulnerability of our work. First, our stories highlight the ethicist's vulnerability experienced in the encounter which is often framed as a moral distress problem to fixed (rather than a constituent element to be explored). Second, even peers and colleagues may radically misunderstand our stories in ways that are detrimental – personally and professionally. Clinical experiences exceed the *still widely varied* studying, training, and frameworks established in the field and so we have to grapple with differences in our own and each other's clinical practice in sustained and public engagement, exploring what all matters in the work we do, as we each do it, alone, together. Thus, in Part III, the narratives in the following two chapters take up and take seriously these challenges and risks, illustrating the element of vulnerability in clinical ethics work, and considering storytelling itself as an element of practice.

## Notes

1  Finder, Stuart G. and Bliton, Mark J. (2011). Responsibility after the apparent end: 'Following-up' in clinical ethics consultation. *Bioethics* 25 (7):413–424.
2  Pirsig, Robert M. (1974). *Zen and the Art of Motorcycle Maintenance*. New York: Bantam Books, 1981 edition. pp. 4–5.
3  *Ibid.*
4  Finder, Stuart G. and Mark J. Bliton (eds.) (2018). *Peer Review, Peer Education, and Modeling in the Practice of Clinical Ethics Consultation: The Zadeh Project*. Springer Verlag.
5  Finder, Stuart G. (2018). The Zadeh Scenario. In Stuart G. Finder and Mark J. Bliton (eds.), *Peer Review, Peer Education, and Modeling in the Practice of Clinical Ethics Consultation: The Zadeh Project*. Springer Verlag. pp. 21–42.
6  Bliton, Mark J. and Finder, Stuart G. (2018). The Zadeh Project – A Frame for Understanding the Generative Ideas, Formation, and Design. In Stuart G. Finder and Mark J. Bliton (eds.), *Peer Review, Peer Education, and Modeling in the Practice of Clinical Ethics Consultation: The Zadeh Project*. Springer Verlag. pp. 1–18.
7  Finder, Stuart G. and Bliton, Mark J. (2018). Peer Review and Responsibility in/as/for/to Practice. In Stuart G. Finder and Mark J. Bliton (eds.), *Peer Review, Peer Education, and Modeling in the Practice of Clinical Ethics Consultation: The Zadeh Project*. Springer Verlag. pp. 207–228; Zaner, Richard M. (2015). *A Critical Examination of Ethics in Health Care and Biomedical Research: Voices and Visions*. Springer.
8  Bliton and Finder, p. 5.

9  Frolic, Andrea and Rubin, Susan B. (2018). Critical Self-Reflection as Moral Practice: A Collaborative Meditation on Peer Review in Ethics Consultation. In Stuart G. Finder and Mark J. Bliton (eds.), *Peer Review, Peer Education, and Modeling in the Practice of Clinical Ethics Consultation: The Zadeh Project*. Springer Verlag. pp. 47–61.
10  Armstrong, Kelly (2018) Telling About Engagement Is Not Enough: Seeking the "Ethics" of Ethics Consultation in Clinical Ethics Case Reports. In Stuart G. Finder and Mark J. Bliton (eds.), *Peer Review, Peer Education, and Modeling in the Practice of Clinical Ethics Consultation: The Zadeh Project*. Springer Verlag. pp. 63–73.
11  Aulisio, Mark P. (2018). Methodological Lessons for Ethics Consultation. In Stuart G. Finder and Mark J. Bliton (eds.), *Peer Review, Peer Education, and Modeling in the Practice of Clinical Ethics Consultation: The Zadeh Project*. Springer Verlag. pp. 127–137.
12  Rasmussen, Lisa (2018). Standardizing the Case Narrative. In Stuart G. Finder and Mark J. Bliton (eds.), *Peer Review, Peer Education, and Modeling in the Practice of Clinical Ethics Consultation: The Zadeh Project*. Springer Verlag. pp. 151–160.

## Bibliography

Armstrong, Kelly (2018). Telling About Engagement Is Not Enough: Seeking the "Ethics" of Ethics Consultation in Clinical Ethics Case Reports. In Stuart G. Finder and Mark J. Bliton (eds.), *Peer Review, Peer Education, and Modeling in the Practice of Clinical Ethics Consultation: The Zadeh Project*. Cham, Switzerland: Springer Verlag. pp. 63–73.

Aulisio, Mark P. (2018). Methodological Lessons for Ethics Consultation. In Stuart G. Finder and Mark J. Bliton (eds.), *Peer Review, Peer Education, and Modeling in the Practice of Clinical Ethics Consultation: The Zadeh Project*. Cham, Switzerland: Springer Verlag. pp. 127–137.

Bliton, Mark J. and Finder, Stuart G. (2018). The Zadeh Project – A Frame for Understanding the Generative Ideas, Formation, and Design. In Stuart G. Finder and Mark J. Bliton (eds.), *Peer Review, Peer Education, and Modeling in the Practice of Clinical Ethics Consultation: The Zadeh Project*. Cham, Switzerland: Springer Verlag. pp. 1–18.

Finder, Stuart G. (2018). The Zadeh Scenario. In Stuart G. Finder and Mark J. Bliton (eds.), *Peer Review, Peer Education, and Modeling in the Practice of Clinical Ethics Consultation: The Zadeh Project*. Cham, Switzerland: Springer Verlag. pp. 21–42.

Finder, Stuart G. and Bliton, Mark J. (2011). Responsibility after the apparent end: 'Following-up' in clinical ethics consultation. *Bioethics* 25 (7):413–424.

Finder, Stuart G. and Bliton, Mark J. (eds.) ( 2018). *Peer Review, Peer Education, and Modeling in the Practice of Clinical Ethics Consultation: The Zadeh Project*. Cham, Switzerland: Springer Verlag.

Finder, Stuart G. and Bliton, Mark J. (2018). Peer Review and Responsibility in/as/for/to Practice. In Stuart G. Finder and Mark J. Bliton (eds.), *Peer Review, Peer Education, and Modeling in the Practice of Clinical Ethics Consultation: The Zadeh Project*. Cham, Switzerland: Springer Verlag. pp. 207–228.

Frolic, Andrea and Rubin, Susan B. (2018). Critical Self-Reflection as Moral Practice: A Collaborative Meditation on Peer Review in Ethics Consultation. In Stuart G. Finder and Mark J. Bliton (eds.), *Peer Review, Peer Education, and Modeling in the Practice of Clinical Ethics Consultation: The Zadeh Project*. Cham, Switzerland: Springer Verlag. pp. 47–61.

Pirsig, Robert M. (1974). *Zen and the Art of Motorcycle Maintenance*. New York: Bantam Books, 1981 edition.

Rasmussen, Lisa (2018). Standardizing the Case Narrative. In Stuart G. Finder and Mark J. Bliton (eds.), *Peer Review, Peer Education, and Modeling in the Practice of Clinical Ethics Consultation: The Zadeh Project*. Cham, Switzerland: Springer Verlag. pp. 151–160.

# Part III
# Elements of Experience

# 5 Constituent Vulnerability, Constituent Responsibility

**"We Are Power"**

*I.*

She hung herself. Ceci's eight-year-old son found her, almost an hour after she'd excused herself from the dinner table. He had tried to hold her up, but he was only eight and didn't have the strength. Neither did her Grandmother, with whom she and her son lived. The Grandmother held her great-grandson on her lap in her wheelchair while they waited for the paramedics to arrive. And when the EMT holding the body exclaimed that he felt a flutter of a pulse in the neck as his colleagues cut loose the electric cord from the garage ceiling, the Grandmother whispered "Thank God."

*II.*

I met them later – them being Ceci's aunts and cousins and sister and brother-in-law and her pastor. Ceci's Grandmother was at home, kept away by her limited mobility and her great-grandson's care, so the rest of the family was present, meeting with the attending physician in the Intensive Care Unit. This was the second meeting – the attending on service the previous week had told them about the damage to Ceci's brain: the anoxic injury and lack of blood flow, erasing all but the barest, most tenuous of biological function. A week ago, that physician had shown them the MRI scans and explained the way the ventilator was breathing for Ceci almost entirely – but the occasional breath triggering the machine meant Ceci was not "brain dead." The physician was gentle and clear in explaining that for injuries like Ceci's, however, they could tell immediately and could know beyond any medical doubt within a week that Ceci would never wake up again. Then the physician recommended stopping life support: palliative extubation and a plan for comfort-only care until Ceci's death.

Ceci's family understood, or said they did, yet her brother-in-law heard "within a week" to mean that they should continue life support for another 7 days "so that they could be sure." When the ICU attending tried to clarify, to reiterate and insist that they didn't need a full week to prognosticate, the brother-in-law and the sister became insistent themselves, bristling with suspicion, in pugnacious defense of Ceci's chance of improvement. The aunties chimed in, speaking for their mother – Ceci's Grandmother – and Ceci's son, and *their* need to be sure, to have "closure" before withdrawal of the ventilator. And the family's pastor, Pastor Vera, noted they had seen miracles in their community, folks who had been written off as gone, but for whom God still had plans and that His powers that went beyond hope and expectation. Ceci needed to have her week.

DOI: 10.4324/9781003354864-11

### III.

When the social worker, Melissa, sent the text, "Where are you? We need you. Now!," I was walking down the back stairs in the ICU tower, three floors below her unit where Ceci still breathed slightly over the vent. Two days earlier, Melissa had called, concerned that the plan might change as the attending physicians changed service, which could disrupt the tenuous trust that had been established with Ceci's family. The current attending had honored her colleague's acquiescence to Ceci's week of observation, grudgingly, perhaps, but she'd honored it "to the letter." It was now day seven. Since Ceci had not improved, the attending wanted the team to meet with the family to arrange the timing of Ceci's palliative extubation. Melissa had called to say her "spidey-sense" was tingling, and she wanted to give me a "head's up that you might be needed" if the conversation doesn't go well.

It did not go well. When the nurse practitioner had gone into the room to discuss the timing of palliative extubation with the family, Ceci's brother-in-law and sister asked about the most recent scans and wanted to know if there were any changes in Ceci's condition. It had been a week and they needed to know that there hadn't been any improvement before they could "let Ceci go to God."

When the nurse practitioner explained that there hadn't been any more scans because the doctor didn't *need* a scan to see that Ceci was no better, the family was surprised. They calmly and insistently requested that another MRI be done before palliative extubation because *they* needed to know. The nurse practitioner told the attending physician who told the social worker to ask for ethics support. Melissa had dutifully telephoned to update me and to "make the request official from the team." Since then, I had been walking around the hospital on standby, waiting for when team and family were all present.

### IV.

After reading Melissa's text, I turned around and trudged back up the stairs. I arrived on the unit to find Melissa and Dr. Boyard, the current attending, who gave me her own account of the day's events, similar in all the essentials to Melissa's earlier update. She explained that she would try to help the family understand that another scan wasn't indicated: it would not make Ceci's prognosis any clearer to her or to them and so she would not order one. Calmly, and with great sincerity, Dr. Boyard explained that while she understood the distress and need for reassurance and closure, she did not believe in allowing family to dictate medical care. And, it was not reasonable to perform tests that would be treating the family and would not provide any clinical benefit to the patient. "It is my responsibility and my decision to order what is appropriate … or to explain what is not. The scan is not appropriate. It does nothing. It is time to move along, for Ceci's sake." Head inclined, she explained that she hoped Melissa and I could help the family understand. Melissa listened and looked at me, an eyebrow raised.

"Maybe the family just needs to hear it from the doctor, rather than the nurse practitioner," she mused. "They seemed to 'get it': they had a long day of prayer yesterday, with their whole church congregation, and they told me they were at peace, knowing Ceci was at peace. Pastor Vera said, 'She's not even in there – her Spirit is Home, now'."

Melissa continued, tactfully, "Maybe the N.P.'s explanation hadn't been as clear as he thought. Maybe they just need to know *how* the doctors are so sure." Dr. Boyard began to agree: "It's all about trust and it's the family's job to decide whether they trust me to make the appropriate medical decisions."

As Melissa's smile grew stiff, I tried to build on Dr. Boyard's idea, agreeing that trust was crucial and showing ourselves, as the medical team, *to be* trustworthy was even more so: "To be trusted to make the appropriate decisions for each unique person, we should make sure we understood their concerns for Ceci."

Melissa began *a-hem-ing* that the family was waiting to meet the doctor and joked that they were operating with a sense of urgency as strong as Dr. Boyard's, even if for different reasons. We all trooped into the conference room and settled into heavy plastic chairs, disconcerting in their sky-blue cheerfulness.

*V.*

The meeting began as expected – introductions, with Ceci's Grandmother dialed in through speaker-phone, and with the family explaining that they had some questions about the scans. Dr. Boyard acknowledged their questions and explained why, from a medical perspective, she knew beyond doubt that Ceci's injury was irreversible, devastating, and had not changed since the initial scan. She explained that she would not need another scan – clinical observation and correlation with the previous scan was the gold standard in medicine for prognosis with patients like Ceci. It was her responsibility to make these kinds of decisions based on the evidence, and she didn't need any more evidence and, in fact, she could not get any more evidence because there were no additional tests that would show her anything new.

Ceci's brother-in-law began bristling: "So you're saying you won't do the scan? Even though we need to know, even though her grandmother, her son, they need to know? To be sure?"

Dr. Boyard explained again that the scan couldn't add anything: "It would be like x-raying an amputated limb – we know there is nothing there. The first scan showed that there is nothing left of her brain activity – the tissue is dead – it is like the amputated limb."

Pastor Vera began explaining that *while they understood* that her medical knowledge told her so, and that she believed that there hadn't been any change, they and their church had prayed – prayed and fasted and held Ceci up to God – and there might have been some changes because prayer works and God is powerful, and they just needed reassurance. They had seen things before that went against all medical evidence.

Dr. Boyard explained again that she didn't need a scan to know there had been no change because she and her team had examined Ceci every day for a week and, "A scan won't show what you want. I do not have a spiritual MRI. All I can do is use my medical judgment and experience and knowledge and you have to decide whether you trust that or not."

Pastor Vera and Ceci's brother-in-law began talking over each other, and when there was a pause for breath, I interrupted and interjected. I tried reminding everyone that the care team needs patients and families to speak about who the patient is as a person, and what matters to them, including religious concerns, and the physicians are responsible for using this information along with their medical knowledge to make the appropriate medical decisions, including decisions about what kinds of tests or interventions are indicated.

I spoke encouragingly, "So yes, the medical teams trust families to tell us what matters to their loved one so that the doctors can make the best medical plans for *each patient*, and so the families can trust that the doctors are making these plans for this person. *For Ceci.* It is all about trusting each other."

Pastor Vera watched and waited until I took a breath and said: "We just want to know. Can we get the scan or not? Is it *ethical* to refuse a grieving family's request? What does the hospital say about what is ethical, what is *right* to do here?"

That was one of those moments where time thickens – or at least my experience of it does. I saw the challenge in Pastor Vera's eyes. Yes, I did. And, I could sense Dr. Boyard's tension growing, and the family's. Everyone shifting in their seats, bracing themselves for whatever came next. I took a breath, quick and deep, and time flowed as it usually does.

Leaning toward her, my hands open and extended, I replied: "There is not one 'ethical' answer – decisions about what is medically appropriate are clinical judgments – and sometimes they are made on strictly physiologic grounds and sometimes there are other values and considerations at stake as well. Which is why we're trying to understand what it is you are looking for, since the scan you're requesting doesn't give you the kind of reassurance you seem to need. We're having this conversation so we can find out what might help, if the scan isn't the right thing to help ..."

I meant to convey and reaffirm to Dr. Boyard and to the family that ordering the scan was Dr. Boyard's decision and that we were trying to understand both their question and how to help them, and I was trying to figure out how to support Dr. Boyard and the family if this was the medical limit, as it surely appeared to be.

Pastor Vera interrupted again, and all eyes turned to her: "We just need to know what the hospital is going to do now; whether the doctor is going to do this scan. We un-der-*stand* that from medicine, from science, there is no point, that the evidence is clear. But we have seen different evidence – evidence of God's work and God's power and the power of prayer. And we have been praying. We want to see if our prayer had any effect on her brain, anything we could see on the scan because *we've seen that* – in our congregation, in our community. And we want that scan so that if there is no change, we can go forward, knowing we have done everything we could, given her every chance. So, we want to know. If you tell us we cannot have that scan, well, we will still want it, but we'll have tried and pushed for it. And even if we can't have it, at least we'll know we tried and we'll live with that. We'll have to adjust to that."

## VI.

As this measured but insistent plea rolled to its end, Ceci's family turned their gazes from Pastor Vera's face to Dr. Boyard's and my eyes followed theirs. I had heard the opening – the moment of their recognition and acceptance of Dr. Boyard's decision, even if it was reluctant and resigned. I waited to hear the final – "No, I'm sorry, but the scan is not indicated and I will not order something that's not medically appropriate" – from this physician. My thoughts raced ahead toward how to support the family in their disappointment and resignation, to affirm and support that they had done all they could and asked and pushed and advocated beautifully for Ceci.

"Ok. We'll do the scan. We should have the results tomorrow." And as if her preternaturally calm words were a hammer release, Dr. Boyard shot out of the seat and was through the door immediately, her anger lingering like acrid smoke.

## VII.

"She's mad," Pastor Vera observed, looking at me.

My lips tightened and I felt my eyebrow rise as I tried to figure out how to respond, what to say next, while the tension slowly dissipated in the moments after Dr. Boyard's exit. Melissa jumped in, trying to put an ameliorative frame on Dr. Boyard's abrupt departure: that she was a doctor who listened and that she must have heard what they were asking, that Pastor Vera had done such a good job of expressing and describing their faith and the closure the MRI would provide. Ceci's brother-in-law and the aunties nodded, but Pastor Vera looked as skeptical as I felt. Trying to support Melissa's efforts, and to figure out what my next steps might be, now that Dr. Boyard had agreed so abruptly to the scan, I asked them if they could tell me a bit more about their tradition and what they were seeking. It felt anticlimactic, but somehow necessary to ask. I explained that if I could understand a bit more about where they were coming from, it could help me learn how to help other families in the future. I listened as Pastor Vera began describing a biblically literal, born-again, Christ-bearing, evangelical, Pentecostal church, but my mind wandered when her description started ringing familiar bells from my Southern roots – I'd heard this hymn and knew the high notes. I realized that I wasn't going to need to support the family as I had imagined – they had all the support they needed from the Spirit and the Saints, on earth and in Heaven. My mind kept casting about as Pastor Vera gave examples of others in their church "who had been declared brain dead and woke up – after prayer, after fasting! They were fine!" So was Ceci's family. This experience fit in with others they knew: no matter what the scan showed, Spirit, God's power triumphed in this room today.

It occurred to me, thinking about what had just happened, that Dr. Boyard might need the support instead. I was still stunned by Dr. Boyard's decision, and her anger, which had flashed and burned so unexpectedly, so palpably. I worried that *she* might need support because she might not have felt supported – by me. Maybe she heard my invitation to the family to speak as "siding with them," or saw my acknowledgement of "other considerations" as forcing her into a corner and she was angry, feeling powerless. Or maybe she was just tired of the conversation, when she realized how long exploring what they needed could take. I wasn't sure what she was thinking but I knew I needed to find her before I left the unit, to see if I could find out. I needed to see if I could understand the roots of her rage, if I could get her to tell me what happened. I was not looking forward to that conversation, but I couldn't put it off any longer.

I dragged my attention back to Ceci's family and to Pastor Vera, to the ebullience of their praise. Thanking them for sharing the story of their faith and the reasons behind their request. I echoed Melissa's reassurance, without believing it for a minute, that this conversation may have helped Ceci's physician understand some of the non-medical things that mattered in taking care of her.

"The spirit is powerful and we are Spirit," said Pastor Vera. "We are Power." And Ceci's brother-in-law, sisters, and aunties nodded, "Amen." While through the speaker-phone came her Grandmother's fervent, "Thank God."

### Afterwards/After Words

"I feel raped. Raped. I'm sorry, but it's true. I feel completely violated."

Her words were flying daggers. "I was just forced to do something that goes against all my training and experience and how I'm supposed to take care of people. Against everything I am as a physician. It is unconscionable for them to put me into this kind of a position, where if I don't give in to their demands, I am the bad guy. Especially if they're religious. But medicine can't meet their religious demands for proof. I don't *have* a spiritual MRI. There's just no way out for me. It's unconscionable to do the scan – I think it's fraud – insurance fraud! – and malpractice! Because it doesn't do anything but treat this family's grief but if I don't do it, they are angry and feel cheated and discriminated against. And so yes, I feel like I've been *raped* when families like this push it all onto me."

I sat in her office as she paced the floor. I listened to her talk, struggling to understand and trying to work past her language of rape and victimhood to what was underneath. She was trying to give voice to the *something* embodied in her anger at the family's request and her own decision to order the scan and I needed to understand what that was.

"How am I supposed to practice when families can make such demands, especially in the hospital? Science and medicine are clear – were clear a week ago! – what her outcome would be and she is *suffering* on that ventilator. We're *making* her suffer because this family is grieving, and they think another scan is going to fix that. It's not and it just makes Ceci suffer longer. And now *I'm* the one doing that to her. I'm not able to practice good medicine, to take care of Ceci *properly*, because they're making me use medicine and technology to treat *their* grief. Not Ceci – *them*. And because of religion, I can't say 'No.' It's offensive." She spat the word.

I listened, trying to hear. We reviewed different aspects of the conversation – a debrief as I often try to do with the team or family, or sometimes both. After all, I can't be sure I've understood them, or that they understood each other, or that a moment's understanding stays stable, takes root. And sometimes, as happened in Dr. Boyard's office, more gets said about what matters: the "cruel radiance of what is"[1] becomes clearer and emerges from the unsaid. Boyard and I got a little clearer, together, alone. Although we talked again about the frames of physician responsibility and family responsibility, she still insisted that "these families" were unreasonable in making the demands at all. I listened, and we reflected on the challenges of caring for patients who are parts of families, left behind to grieve after a death. Eventually her pacing slowed and her tone quieted.

We sat, for a moment, in the sadness of this young woman's approaching death, set in motion a week ago when she went out to her garage.

I was relieved, when I left, that Boyard's rage had dissipated as we talked, relieved that it hadn't seemed to be directed at me. Yet as I left and thought more about our conversation and the family meeting, the more puzzled I became. What happened here, and what am I to learn from it? What am I supposed to do?

### Vulnerability and Responsibility in Clinical Ethics: Connections and Reflections with Hoffmaster, Spiegelberg, and Zaner

"The Spirit is powerful and we are Spirit."
"I feel completely violated. There's just no way out for me."
"I was still stunned ... I needed to see if I could understand."
"It just makes Ceci suffer more ... and now I'm the one doing that to her."
"What is the ethical thing to do here?"

I am still living through the memories captured in this story. Not the actual moments of indecision and uncertainty about getting a scan for Ceci in those days and hours before her death. Rather, it's more the learning, if I could call it that, that flows out of those experiences of uncertainty, the deep and compelling need to understand, wondering how to interpret shifting dynamics of power when those meanings seem to appear and then recede into something else, and in all that, my own awareness of vulnerability and responsibility remain. There is, to be sure, some power in all that.

There are any number of elements of responsibility in this story to isolate and think about – especially referring back to those that have been reviewed in previous chapters – disruption and attention, ethics as self-reflection and self-education, the need for affiliation and attunement. Here, I'm going to focus on the overwhelming and overlapping experiences of vulnerability and responsibility that are active, lively, and exemplified in this encounter. Vulnerability was not (and is not) a stable category description, but a complex experience, shared by those involved in the particular circumstances of Ceci's devastating neurological injury.

The deep link between vulnerability and responsibility is one of the most important recognitions I carried out of the ICU that day after my conversations with the clinicians, in the family meeting, with the physician afterwards, in her office. And in the years since, trying to think through and understand that kind of vulnerability and the responsibility it demands has led to some reflections that continue to shape my practice. Everyone in that story experienced and demonstrated their own unique and connected vulnerabilities and responsibilities, which allows this story to serve as an example of those connections in clinical ethics encounters – and hence clinical ethics practice.

Quite often when ethicists talk about vulnerability, they focus on patients of families, or those made vulnerable by disease, disabilities, and health disparities. The presumption is that those in positions of limited power are vulnerable to those in positions of power. While not inaccurate in many cases, the encounter with Ceci's family and care team drove home the idea of vulnerability as shared among anyone involved in a clinical ethics consultation (including the clinical ethics consultant!). Specifically: a person experiences vulnerability by simple fact of being in a deeply uncertain moral experience that they did not choose to face, do not necessarily want to engage, and find themselves confronted with the reality of being responsible for words, choices, actions, and decisions. Everyone may have their own vulnerabilities that they bring into the situation, due to social factors like race, gender, education, power and authority, etc., but *this* vulnerability of unchosen, urgent unknowing is shared in the taken-for-granted characteristics of everyday life, so it can easily go without notice. The shared vulnerability of being caught in a moment of real, live choice is urgent, unavoidable, and overwhelming – especially where one's choices and actions look to be deeply relevant to the outcomes, aftermaths, and even future choices, i.e., where one's response matters.[2] The urgent need to know what to choose, to have the uncertainty relieved, the deep hope that one's actions and choices will be right (or at least not wrong), that they'll help (or at least not hurt, not make things worse) connects the inextricable link between vulnerability and responsibility – which stands out as a key element in the clinical experience described above – and in many such moments encountered in clinical ethics work.

### The Dance of Vulnerability and Responsibility

The movement between vulnerability and responsibility has two aspects relevant to clinical ethics consultation. First is the recognition of vulnerability from lack of power and choice, which demands a response from the other. Vulnerability, simply from these others being in such a situation, elicits my notice and may require a response from me as a clinical ethics consultant. Second, that responsibility creates its own vulnerability for the responsible one – for me. That second form is part of what I want to explore here, because it is also intimately related to bearing the weight of and embodying the responsibility for my own engagement with others. Awareness of this movement between a vulnerability that demands my responsibility *and* my responsibility that creates its own vulnerability turns out to be a primary element of responsible practice.

My conversation partners for exploring vulnerability include philosopher and bioethicist, Barry Hoffmaster, phenomenologist Herbert Spiegelberg, and phenomenologist and clinical ethicist, Richard M. Zaner. I learned from Hoffmaster and Zaner by engaging their writings on vulnerability and responsibility in clinical ethics. I draw insights from Spiegelberg's reflections on the existential vulnerability and constituent responsibility shared with other humans. In what follows I'll try to work through these themes to reflect on the experiences with Ceci's family and clinical team and to illustrate the connections between vulnerability and responsibility in clinical ethics work. I want to be extra clear, however, that none of this offers a way out of vulnerability or a way to mitigate it. Rather, the aim is to get clearer about what it is like to be vulnerable, and how to understand and make meaning in experiences of vulnerability as one of the inescapable elements of clinical ethics work.

### Barry Hoffmaster and the Meaning of Vulnerability

Barry Hoffmaster, philosophy professor at the University of Western Ontario and clinical ethicist, published an essay "What does Vulnerability Mean?" in 2006 in the *Hastings Center Report* with several insights that have been helpful both in my clinical practice and in reflecting on practice while writing this book.

Early in the essay, Hoffmaster points out that while the word "vulnerability" is easy to use and used often, it is less often clearly understood. He runs through a variety of dictionary definitions:

vulnerable as being susceptible to something, usually bad; vulnerability as being capable of being physically or emotionally wounded; able to be tempted; to be liable to penalties[3] He notes that none of the typical definitions are particularly helpful for understanding the experiences of or possible meanings of vulnerability because they don't address our multiple and interconnected vulnerabilities. In response to those kinds of limitations, Hoffmaster uses narratives to try to capture the meaning of vulnerability, focusing on descriptors of living with vulnerability or being vulnerable, using examples from his own experiences.[4]

Modeling his own vulnerability as a son and as a clinician, Hoffmaster describes his father's physical, social, emotional, and vulnerability of living for 40 years post-stroke: dependent and limited by "natural causes," and by the social implications that followed. Hoffmaster also draws a related, but different, picture of the vulnerability lived and experienced by his mother in her role as a caregiver for her husband to show the social and emotional wounds and limitations that are uniquely hers, *and* inextricably linked to his. Hoffmaster notes that for the kind of vulnerability associated with "natural causes" there is little if any difference between being vulnerable and being at risk.[5] On the other hand, the vulnerability deriving from "human causes and human creations" includes kinds of vulnerability shaped by impediments in communication and limitations of information available in the circumstances, as well as other cultural factors such as beliefs about the power of medicine. Either or both kinds may be operative in any particular clinical encounter.

Hoffmaster's observations about the vulnerability stemming from "the deeply rooted cultural injunction that associates responsibility with action, rather than just acceptance …"[6] were most relevant to my reflections. He identifies an unspoken but deeply held belief that if someone is "responsible," they will act; if they care, they will *do* something. In looking back at my experiences in the "We Are Power" encounter, that belief emerges as a contributing factor in the vulnerability demonstrated by Ceci's family. They couldn't understand why Dr. Boyard wouldn't just *do* what they asked and get the scan. Didn't she care enough to give them the information they needed? A similar belief seems to have contributed to Dr. Boyard's feelings of vulnerability and conflicted responsibilities, wondering why the family couldn't just take action. Didn't they care enough to end Ceci's suffering?

For Hoffmaster the most important, crucial similarity linking these different types and experiences of vulnerability is "the loss of power that vulnerability imposes and signifies and the attendant loss of control that ensues."[7] He's quite explicit: "We fear vulnerability most immediately because of the particular harms we seek to avoid. But we fear vulnerability most profoundly because of the power we seek to retain."[8] Thinking about my encounter with Ceci's family, we can see their desire to hold the power of making decisions on her behalf and demanding the information they felt they needed for such decisions. And while they anchored their sense of that power in their faith and their authority as her family, their experience of vulnerability was tied to the limitations of that power in a clinical setting, within the institutional expectations and practices of the medical center. On the other hand, we can see Dr. Boyard seeking to retain the power of professional decisions that she saw as her responsibility to make – including power to authorize or rule out diagnostic investigations and therapeutic interventions. Her sense of that sort of power was rooted in her expertise and the authority of medicine and science – which confronted real limits in the face of the faith and authority claimed by Ceci's family.

For Ceci's family and her physician, one aspect of their vulnerability an overlapping (although not shared) sense of being unable to *do something* to help her. More specifically, what keeps them separable is that distinct feeling of being powerless, and that "powerlessness" rooted in an assessment that the other would not *do something* to help her. There is a way to understand that dynamic of vulnerability, in a Hoffmaster quotation from the psychologist Rollo May, where May says, "No human being can stand the perpetually numbing experiences of his own powerlessness."[9] I can imagine that experiences of powerlessness for a family might motivate their strident insistence on information and time before decisions. It strikes me, as well, that repeated experiences of powerlessness might also explain the unexpected rage and angst demonstrated by the physician during and after the conversation.

What I find helpful in this framing is the possibility of recognizing, of naming such experiences of vulnerability in clinical encounters – not to "fix" it or manage it – but to create possibilities for understanding, and to locate possible affiliations and meaning in those experiences. For example, if we shift back toward clinical ethics practice, the quotation from May strikes me as relevant to the clinical ethics consultant and likewise for the field of clinical ethics. In my experience with Ceci's family and team, I had also carried the cultural presumption that being responsible equates to *doing*, and this contributed to my own sense of vulnerability. I found myself suspended in the experience of unknowing, with Ceci's family and with the clinical team – while still fully aware that my own sense of responsibility and the presumed authority of my role could easily push me to act *in reaction* to my own and others' expectation that to *care* meant to *act*.

Hoffmaster asks, then answers, a crucial question here: "How do we respond to such sweeping debilitating vulnerability? Vulnerability gives us much to fear and we respond to it as we do to other fears: we tried to suppress and ignore it."[10] Reflecting back, I can see that, in those moments of shared unknowing in the conversation, I became acutely aware of an unwelcome power: that I could eliminate the fear of others' uncertainty, the experience of not-knowing, with a "nudge." I could have answered Pastor' Vera's question about whether it was "ethical" to refuse a grieving family's request. Either answer – yes or no – would have ended the conversation and closed down the question. With my "authorization," I could have explained a choice in a way that removed from others the presumed responsibility to act: I could leave them only the need to accept. Yet, as I understood and still understand, choosing-for-others was not my responsibility. Choosing-for-others harbors its own impediments and harms, for me, and for them. One aspect of responsibility that becomes clear was my need to resist the impulse to suppress or mitigate the shared experience of vulnerability, and thus, to remain in that space of limbo and unknowing with the family and care team. That was *my* responsibility. Which also meant living in and with the recognition of the limits to my responsibility: living with my own vulnerability and experiencing those limits.

### *Clinical Ethics Consultant's Responsibility to Vulnerability*

I'm telling (and retelling) the "We Are Power" story as an example, an occasion to consider how ethics consultants might respond in the face of repeated encounters with our own vulnerability – evoked by and linked to our responsibilities as clinical ethics consultants. The default of associating responsibility with action can make taking up the mantle of expertise and donning the armor of authority seem appealing. We ethicists can get clear frameworks for analysis! We can rescue others from their distress! We can nudge people to the better answer! We have consensus! We can resolve the tensions and help people find closure! All of these impulses and ideas are present within the literature as solutions to the problem of vulnerability – especially to ours as ethics consultants encountering the vulnerability of patients, families, and providers. These voices seem to be whispering (or shrieking) the same thing: if we are experts, authorities, action-bound, then we won't have to take into account such disorienting moments in these deeply uncertain moral encounters.

The story of my encounter with Ceci's family and clinical team demonstrates just how insufficient and ineffective are the efforts toward denying or escaping vulnerability. Along with Hoffmaster (and echoed in Spiegelberg and Zaner, below), I see vulnerability as a source of our concern for others and also a source for our interest in and reliance on others. We are all vulnerable by nature of our embodied humanity and vulnerable both from "natural causes" and social, cultural, and interpersonal causes. Hoffmaster points out that "all human beings are born into vulnerability and remain deeply vulnerable for some time ... Moreover, our universal vulnerability resonates with a moral significance ...: it is our very vulnerability that creates the need for morality."[11] Shared vulnerability is the moral basis for caring for others' vulnerability, although Hoffmaster also acknowledges that vulnerability and morality aren't always tied together for well-articulated reasons: i.e., since vulnerability is antithetical to the myth of western individualism, because moral philosophy typically ignores the body in favor of the idealized, rational mind, and because vulnerability engages our feelings as much as our minds and such feelings are also rarely welcome in the western philosophical traditions.[12]

That said, when we recognize the depth and breadth of our vulnerabilities, "we realize how much we need the help of others to protect us from our weaknesses and our infirmities,"[13] and even further, as Hoffmaster insists, how much the vulnerable person is capable of making us feel. We can feel compassion for that person's losses and that person's suffering. We can also feel our common humanity – our own fragility in our own dependence. If we do, we truly can care for that person and for ourselves. That is what vulnerability means for us.[14]

Hoffmaster's emphasis on inherent vulnerability, tied to shared human experience as the basis for responsibility strikes a deep chord in my clinical practice.

I read Hoffmaster's essay around the same time as my experiences with women and partners considering maternal-fetal surgery to repair spina bifida in the MOMS trial and it helped to make clear the kinds of vulnerability that demand care and generate care. As then, so with the "We Are Power" encounter with Ceci's family, Pastor Vera, and Dr. Boyard, years later. That encounter brings the connection between vulnerability and responsibility into even more crystalline focus, which resonated through another essay from over 30 years prior – encountered during my training and revisited on a semi-regular basis ever since.

Herbert Spiegelberg's 1974 essay, "Ethics for Fellows in the Fate of Existence,"[15] was republished in a 1986 collection entitled, *Steppingstones towards an Ethics for Fellow Existers: Essays 1944–1983* and it lays out what Spiegelberg came to understand about responsibility and ethics in human experience. Writing as a philosopher and phenomenologist, and as a human who had experienced disruptions of war from childhood throughout the 20th century, Spiegelberg's essay aims to account for both the unchosen fate that unites human beings as fellows in existence, and the obligations – the responsibilities – these fated circumstances demand. The themes he identifies and articulates echo down through my clinical experiences – including that encounter with Ceci and her family and care team – all of us, present without control in that moment.

### Herbert Spiegelberg's Ethics for Fellow Existers

When thinking about the challenges and choices that emerge in clinical encounters and the weight of that uncertainty, Herbert Spiegelberg provides several helpful ways to articulate the un-chosenness of each of our lives. This universal experience in human life – at the most basic level, whatever other choices or opportunities may emerge – for Spiegelberg, is what binds us in a shared vulnerability and demands of us a shared responsibility.

Spiegelberg starts by noting "the inexorableness of fate as the prime and ultimate fact of our being" and chooses the word "fate" to emphasize that

> the victims of this fate are totally ignorant of any possible meaning in it or purpose behind it. In this sense the mere fact of our existence is something that has befallen us, has happened to us as an 'accident' in a sense which does not imply a denial of cause.[16]

No one asks to be born (or "worlded" as Zaner writes later)[17]; and yet the lack of our own control over being born, our existence, is the one thing undeniably linking humans to each other. Spiegelberg recommends "we had better face our situation and in fact our predicament soberly without such futile emotions as cosmic rage or exultation."[18] Our shared, unchosen "predicament" creates the fellowship that is the source of our bond with and responsibility to each other.

For Spiegelberg the term "fellowship" is less fraught, less sexist, and less theologically loaded than "brotherhood" and offers more substance and seriousness than "fellow feeling" or the idea of voluntary association. He argues that the idea of "being caught in the same unchosen predicament" holds a broader and more valid claim as a bond among and between other humans.[19] Fellowship, though, can only make sense in the context of something shared by or among persons considered to be "fellows" and Spiegelberg moves quickly past vague and even trivial or shallow connections – "same-fated" or "fate-joined" fellows linked by sharing a country or a time in history. He defines "like-fated" or "parallel-fated" fellowship as sharing characteristics that are similar, but parallel without real, direct connection – sex, or skin color, or class. While Spiegelberg outlines several examples of parallel-fate that can be the basis for fellowship, he notes these are limited because they are particular to some and not all. What connects every human is the shared fate of existing as a human. It is here that he sees a shared bond that creates an ethical obligation to our fellow existers.[20]

Spiegelberg argues that despite sharing this most basic feature of our existence, we are not always aware of this kind of fellowship, these kinds of connections: "to make us conscious of them takes comparing, pointing out, even awakening. No wonder we are so little aware of our fellowship in the fate of existence."[21] He observes that it is much easier to imagine and accept ethical obligations to "fate-joined fellows" linked by the accidents such as country of birth or time in history than our broader connection as fellow existers. Similarly, while we also may feel fellowship with those "like-fated" others of shared race, sex, class, etc., recognizing our obligations to fellow existers requires an "ethical awakening" by taking seriously what he calls "the accident of birth," The fact that none of us have a choice about being born, or with what body, attributes and abilities or challenges, or into what circumstances, resources, communities, or even time or era. The accident of birth is the one thing that connects all humans, per Spiegelberg, because it "assigns to each one of us a specific lot and no other. To take the phrase seriously is, I firmly believe, the lever which can finally move the dead weight of our social lethargy."[22]

Spiegelberg wants people to acknowledge that we need "a new approach to ethics [which] tries to make us face the fact of our existence in all its inexorableness, cosmically and morally,"[23] and to do so as a way to claim a realistic concept of "existential justice (and injustice)." He observes that everyone is born into the world without choice – cast into a fate and an accident of birth without consent, which Spiegelberg argues is an existential wrong in principle (and practice). He writes,

> the future of one's own very self-being involves essentially an existential wrong in the sense of a 'slight' to one's basic freedoms. There is something morally incongruous about the lack of consent to one's own basic being. There is perhaps even an essential indignity to this predicament.[24]

Since no human can say "No" to their fate of existence, for Spiegelberg, their being "exposed to being is a 'condemnation' without prior hearing" and means that the self begins as an innocent victim.[25] The affront to freedom continues, for Spiegelberg, by recognizing that the exister had no choice about any of the given elements of that existence – neither being a human (versus a tree or a cat or a mountain) nor any of the particulars of sex, race, temperament, appearance, or gifts or "disabilities" has any essential let alone morally necessary relation relative to that self.[26] This is further confirmed by our lack of choice in being born into our initial station (historical time, national, cultural, or social situation). Such accidental factors contribute to what Spiegelberg calls "an essential moral imbalance in being born into any such station" whether one of power and privilege or one of deep lack and destitution. Even more explicitly: "there is no moral basis for and no excuse for pride and shame over congenital conditions which are all accidents of birth."[27]

Rather, Spiegelberg roots ethics in our obligation to others *because* of our shared injustice of being thrown into the world and thrown into our lives without choice. For Spiegelberg there are "moral imbalances" that need to be called out, and these occur when people share similar situations but are "subject to a discrimination which favors those more "'fortunate' by the mere 'happenstance' and disfavors the 'unfortunate' victims of 'bad luck'."[28] There is something "basically wrong about such a fate and what is more something ought to be done about it,"[29] which grounds Spiegelberg's belief that fellow human beings are tied, by the similar fates of their very being, to each other and to the demand for a compensatory existential justice: unearned advantages call for redress.

To achieve or even have the possibility of working toward realizing such demands, Spiegelberg maintains that we must put ourselves "vicariously into the places of our fellow beings, whether privileged or handicapped" to have any chance of understanding what it means for them to "experience their fates and make appropriate amends."[30] Here, Spiegelberg resonates with Hoffmaster's need to explore the meanings, rather than the definitions of vulnerability. Spiegelberg also provides a grounding to understand the moral orders created by the affiliation with human distress and the recognition of multiple voices in the attunements described by Richard Zaner and Pierre Bourdieu: understanding and meaning are dependent upon imaginative and careful attention to the other. Spiegelberg sees the affiliation created by actions of imaginative self-transposal, and the need for *being* understanding, as a duty generated from the accident of birth and the injustice of that existential imbalance. Or, in perhaps my favorite line of the essay: "The fact of the 'accident' of our congenital 'nature' calls for a primal tolerance for and patience with one another's natures ... none of us has earned his endowment or lack of it."[31] I could add "primal tolerance" to an ethics' consultants job requirement without a moment's hesitation.

In the end, Spiegelberg shifts away from the imbalance of the accidents of birth (class, religion, family structure, as well as nationality, sex, gender, race, and gifts or disabilities) that are unevenly distributed. He reiterates the fact of our existence as the basic fellowship behind all of them, which creates a need for action. Spiegelberg's fellowship invites "the realization both in the sense of insight and of actualization in practice": to approach every human being as a being who has been cast into their lot without their own doing; to consider all human beings as fellow victims of a morally unaccountable fate; and to treat every human person as a new being in their own right.[32] This requires, for Spiegelberg, an imaginative transposal into the plight of the other and a patience, compassion, and mercy to both the other and to ourselves. In doing so Spiegelberg offers hope:

> the way from chance to choice is the path of human reclamation of 'a universe we never made.' Hence, we ought to consider human beings not only as fellow victims of the accidents of birth but also fellow agents capable of accepting or rejecting this fate by converting their congenital endowments into a new order based on choice.[33]

The vulnerability of existence – unchosen and unjustifiable – creates possibilities for empowerment through choice and action in response to the unchosen vulnerabilities we all experience.[34] This possibility of responsibility – *the call to be responsible* to and for those equally suffering under the fate of existence – also draws attention to the other unchosen fates that people bear.

*The Undeserved Unfairness of Happenstance in Clinical Encounters*

Spiegelberg resonates in my clinical practice because that universal current of chance and happenstance becomes almost shocking in clinical settings – no matter what the context. Chance and happenstance – revealed in the infinite variety of illness and injury to which humans are susceptible – are also clearly visible in the equally vast and wildly combined array of characteristics that shape each human in their "unchosen lot": the race or gender, the religious traditions or social class that undergird their experiences of illness and injury, caring for others, and being cared for by others.

Spiegelberg's frame of un-chosenness, the vulnerability inherent in being fated to the particular community, family, the *body* we occupy, helps to illustrate, to depict, and remind me that part of the clinical ethics work is to help people identify the uniqueness of their positions and perspectives, and that work is necessary to participate in creating the possibilities for Spiegelberg's "imaginative transposal" in clinical ethics encounters. I had no expectation of ever getting Pastor Vera and Ceci's family to accept the roots of Dr. Boyard's knowing, nor that she would start to share their belief. I focused on creating a space, modeling and constructing a possibility for them to hear the other's perspectives,[35] and to do that I needed to listen for any possibilities of overlap in their stories, for some room to maneuver from the positions each held so tightly. Participating as the ethics consultant, part of my responsibility was to be attentive to and attuned to the various vulnerabilities people carried and displayed (or tried to hide); to try to see and hear the needs and the demands of these others in front of me, caught in their moments.

None of them choose to be in that particular clinical moment, in that interaction with each other – any more than they choose their race or gender. Even the choices of association and intention that contributed to everyone's presence were only potential contributions to the encounter: Pastor Vera as the family's clergyperson, Dr. Boyard in her choices to pursue medicine, me in my choices that led to my clinical ethics work. We were all subsumed in an enclave of the chance of *this* encounter, *this* contingent affiliation and engagement. We all shared *that* vulnerability – and struggled to choose and act responsively and hence responsibly in that moment.

Reflecting on these vulnerabilities and responsibilities in clinical ethics practice, and how deeply entwined they are, I would mention that as times goes on, I am more appreciative of the convergences and connections between these themes in others' thought that preceded my own. In particular, I am grateful to Spiegelberg for the recognition of the vulnerability we share in the fellowship of existers, and the questions of how to respond to that vulnerability.

The weight of responsibility that emerges in a clinical ethics encounter, the oft-referenced phrase of an "entrustable profession," has sharp teeth in clinical ethics work where actions, words, and choices can profoundly shape meanings and options. The obligation to respond does not guarantee a response, as anyone who has found themselves responsible in a clinical context knows: neither we nor those around us rise to every occasion or give all in every encounter. Our responsibility always exceeds our ability. The vulnerability of the Other always demands more than we can give. But our limits don't diminish the call or the weight of responsibility, which is how we experience our own vulnerability.

Nor, as Spiegelberg's reflections drive home, do we get to choose to whom we are responsible, or to choose who is vulnerable. In clinical ethics work, the one in most need is often – but not always – the patient. The vulnerable may include someone not typically considered vulnerable – a clinician, patient's family, or ethics consultant. Neither responsibility nor vulnerability are singular: they are movements and they generate meaning, and they shift and change with even a "single" consultation. In any given consultation, the responsibility to the situation means the ethics consultant's responsibility and service to one participant might be, and often is, mitigated and minimized by the demand of yet another. The multiple participants expand questions about the ethics consultant's obligations into a question of justice: what am I to do in service to more than one? Especially if it is one I would not choose (if I had choice)? This emergence of justice is particularly striking and helpful when thinking about vulnerability in a clinical context because there are always multiple others with demands and needs, with their own devastating vulnerability. In the clinical encounter, the healthcare professional is always directed to be responsible to the one who presents in need. At the same time, there are always more persons involved who are in need – and each demands a response.

The experience captured in "We Are Power" highlights this unchosen and unexpected responsibility of the self for the other, and a more detailed reflection may illustrate these points for clinical ethics practice. In the story I came into the situation in the middle of an unfolding dynamic – already responsible to that situation because of my role as clinical ethics consultant. I encountered different individuals, each with some expectations of what I might do or how I might help. And, some of those expectations were different from the ones held by those who requested clinical ethics consultation, and from those who entered the conversation and learned that "ethics has been consulted." I knew I was responsible for my actions and words and choices in my role as the ethics consultant. And yet … as the conversation became thick and heavy, there was a kind of responsibility that became located in me, *as mine*.

In the midst of the conversation, pinballing around the room, I saw the faces of the others emerge in their clear demand: Pastor Vera speaking as the face and voice of Ceci and her family, with their desperate demand to know, their pain raw and their hope, militant and faithful. Their vulnerability and despair called for surcease on *their* terms, the ethical demand was for what met their needs. As the ethics consultant I felt shattered against this demand, because it went against what is typically understood as appropriate within the clinical frame and domains of diagnostics and therapeutics. After all, the physician was 100% right in seeing that the demand for imaging as nonsensical in terms of changing Ceci's care plan. And because her responsibility included developing a clinical plan – that might include drawing limits based on the pathophysiology and prognosis. I thought I was making space in the conversation to help Dr. Boyard articulate the clinical frames and options available or not – after all, that was the gist of her request for consultation. And yet I found myself fully surrendered in a moment of *justice* – faced with Ceci – represented by her grieving family and eloquent pastor *and* by Dr. Boyard in her frustrated bewilderment.

I knew these moments were significant and also fragile, shifting in the sense that several moral orders were in play and circulating around each other. I was acutely aware of the need and vulnerability that girded the family's request, and what was demanded was a response that exceeded the rational, the medically appropriate, the institutionally justifiable approach. And yet, there was an *ethical* response demanded by and for the individual in front of me, Ceci, this moral obligation to the other in need, laid bare and raw. At the same time, I was acutely aware of the need and the vulnerability of the physician. She faced an impossible demand and bore the weight of the "No" expected from her role as an intensivist, her institutional obligations, and her professional responsibility to her patient in the hospital bed. Dr. Boyard's recognition of that responsibility's weight and seriousness, her moral obligation to act within the best and highest of her skill, knowledge, and practice somehow was expressed as spirit-crushing in this moment because those are formed within operational norms of rationality so dominant in our bureaucratic systems of health care. Those hollowed out institutional and professional frames now came into direct contact with the ways that these operational formats and norms were indifferent to individuals, like Ceci and her family, and yet, Dr. Boyard was nonetheless responsible. Her responsibility was experienced personally and enacted interpersonally in a way that evoked her own exposure to what she believed was the "source" of her authority: she was also deeply vulnerable and in need of a response.

Finally, I recognized my own vulnerability. I could see myself as a fellow exister in this moment, differentiated from the self who walked in as a clinical ethics consultant. I struggled in the perilous quicksand of suspecting that I could push the conversation in one direction or another. I could take on the responsibility for others, including their responsibility: I could voice a "No," claiming an authority from my position as ethics "expert," which could shut down the demands of the family, even if it did not address their vulnerability or their grief, neither current nor future. Or I could shut down the physician's protest against further imaging by speaking a "Yes" with the same kind of claimed authority, with any number of justifications based on previous agreements or understandings about what was good for the family or good for the patient. In surrender – sharing others' unknowing, I was suspended amid appeals to justice, convicted by my overwhelming responsibility to both needs, un-meet-able for each without harm to the other.

The vulnerabilities and responsibilities demonstrated by Paster Vera and Ceci's family, as well as Dr. Boyard, were part of who they were: Pastor Vera and the family's responsibilities to push and pray; Dr. Boyard's responsibility to make scientifically and medically backed decisions, based on her medical expertise and knowledge. Similarly, I was there by the circumstances of my role, which was now exceeded, and I remained there with my own commitments which may not be relevant to these others. I trembled in the shifting moments of believing I was responsible to those faces in front of me – each also responsible and working out *in real time* (suspended, unspeakable, nearly intolerable moral time) the question of what was to be done, in the face of such vulnerability and distress.

Any number of retrospective arguments could be made that, as an ethics consultant, I failed in my responsibility by not making a clear recommendation and argument for not answering Pastor Vera's most pointed question of "What's the ethical thing to do?" For instance, taking up the frame of responsibility to the single other in front of me, I failed, because in fact I refused responsibility for the demands of the devastated vulnerable one about whom Vera asked that question: for Ceci. And yet, it wasn't clear whether that "vulnerable" one was Ceci, or Vera, since Ceci "was going to God" … and, thinking about the multiple others present in that moment, I was caught in an absolute responsibility to all of them, in my role and as my own responsible, fellow-existing self, trying to hold that space open to see what actual moral order emerged from the overlap and interactions of the ones already in play.

Vulnerability and responsibility do, however, elicit responses, actions, and in that moment, Dr. Boyard burst out with *her* response to Ceci's family – to their devastated demand, their grieving, vulnerable need-to-know. Her response – unwilling, perhaps unchosen – and yet stemming from *her* responsibility, released *my* responsibility by creating a moment of certainty: for that moment, there was no longer a multitude of faces with competing demands for my response. But when she left abruptly while the social worker and I tried to wrap up conversation with Ceci's family, her echoing absence left another demand, another plea from a place of devastation and vulnerability. I found myself reacting to Dr. Boyard's distress, her need and vulnerability and wondering how I could respond while I was still reeling from this encounter with Ceci's family and Pastor Vera, still stumbling through the recoil of the momentary holding in absolute responsibility that defaulted to a hollowed out norm, "do what the family wants." I wondered if Dr. Boyard's rough departure, her reaction in that clinical ethics encounter had something to do with my involvement, or was made more difficult by my actions or inactions. Her reaction to owning up to her responsibility evoked questions about my own professional responsibility, now, to her. And still, I found myself without a clear answer for the experiential question: "What am I to do now?"

### *Richard M. Zaner's Meditation on Vulnerability*

For considering this kind of vulnerability in a clinical context, Richard Zaner's work is once again instructive and relevant. In particular, in 2000, Zaner published an essay in *Medicine, Health, & Philosophy,* entitled "Power and Hope in the Clinical Encounter: A Meditation on Vulnerability," that explores the element of vulnerability as it shapes responsibility in clinical ethics practice.[36] Zaner uses a clinical experience, told in shards and snippets, from overview to down-in-it detail, to explore, identify, give an account of, and reflect on key elements of such clinical encounters. Zaner focuses on vulnerability through kaleidoscopic twists of contributing lenses: the Asclepius myth that roots the Hippocratic imperative to do no harm and to care for the vulnerable, countered by the Gyges myth to ask: what keeps humans from taking advantage when they are in positions of power? He also incorporates insights from philosophers Alfred Schutz, Kurt Wolff, and Herbert Spiegelberg to emphasize different aspects of the clinical relationships marked by vulnerability and responsibility, which are both opened by and oriented by the dialogues that emerge in clinical encounters.

In the story he tells of encountering a patient, Ms. Oland, Zaner reflects on the connection he felt in the encounter, though Mrs. Oland' awareness and interaction was limited even at best. Zaner writes,

> She and I are face-to-face with each other; she within her history, her still unfolding biography, me within mine. At first though, this mutual presence is only a sort of promise which might or might not be fulfilled … an orientation … that invites each of us to participate in the other's biography and history …[37]

This recognition of the relationship that exists and is constituted by the mere encounter parallels Spiegelberg's insistence that we are all fellows in the fate of existence, obligated to each other. Here Zaner eloquently describes the inequality of that relationship – that the patient, the vulnerable one, i*n her very vulnerability* ought to dictate the moral dynamics of the encounter. She commands the room, demands the response Zaner finds himself giving: absolute attention and care. He explains

> I noticed straight away that everything in the room is arranged in a very specific and powerful way with respect to *her*. *She* is the center; everything in the room is there for *her*, She is the focus for all the equipment, activity, procedures, and for anyone who comes in (nurse, doctors, family, visitors).[38]

Her presence and her needs demand attention and care, responsive awareness of her, as she is lying in the bed. In the experience shared in the "We Are Power" story, although the patient herself, Ceci, was absent from the room, I recall a similar energy and attention, with Ceci's family and Pastor Vera participating in her vulnerability – her demand for care – which calls for what Zaner describes as a kind of decentering: "here, 'you' and 'I' matter far less than she, talk thus centers on and around and regarding her: she is 'that-with-which-respect-to-whom' the room is organized at this moment."[39] Zaner notes, like Hoffmaster, that both the experiential physiologic limitations and the changes in social relationships contribute to the patient's vulnerability – "utterly exposed to gazes, touches, voices, not to mention the far more intrusive 'interventions' common to most medical encounters."[40] The deep asymmetry in her relationships with other people and to herself in her body, in the world, creates an existential vulnerability.

For Zaner the myth of Asclepius illustrates one response to this vulnerability: taking care, being careful, holding oneself restrained and responsible for the person who is so limited by circumstance and happenstance. This deep vulnerability calls to the healers of Asclepius, to take on "certain fundamental responsibilities" motivated by philanthropy (love for the fellow human) including responsibility to "turn his attention to himself, to heal himself before trying to heal others …"[41] In reading Zaner, I hear parallels to Hoffmaster's stories of his father's "natural causes" of vulnerability, but also the vulnerability experienced by Hoffmaster's mother: her not-knowing, her guilt, and her inability to do what she felt obligated to do for her husband.

Zaner also explores a second response available in the encounter with the vulnerable other – the path of Gyges who, per Plato's myth, lies, seduces, and kills his way to power in the Kingdom using a magic ring that cloaks the wearer in invisibility, i.e., that shields the wearer from responsibility.[42] Zaner asks and is troubled by what he calls "the ancient enigma" of wondering what could prompt a healer (or any human) to not take advantage of the vulnerable other in that face-to-face encounter. He writes,

> the clinical encounter is haunted by the figure of Gyges and its temptations to manipulation, control, or otherwise taking advantage of the ineluctably vulnerable person. In the interplay of these mythic images, the moral character of encountering the other as ill may best be understood. Why Hippocrates and not Gyges?[43]

Here, responsibility for not taking advantage, for keeping the trust unavoidably offered by the vulnerable other, with their all-encompassing, compelling need, is in the hands of the less vulnerable people. Zaner describes the vulnerable Ms. Oland as "a center of gravity, pulling others' looks, gestures, and words towards her,"[44] demanding a response of care and attention, pointing out the power of vulnerability in what Hoffmaster calls "exposure to risk." Zaner writes,

> That very exposure is morally commanding and I sensed it immediately on entering her room. Don't touch anything! Watch what you say! Note how potent her vulnerability is: it attracts, directs anyone who approaches to be careful in what is said and done. A need to be restrained yet concerned silently governs, just because she is, so to speak, so vulnerable. Her exposure to others' actions and words augers caution, compels attentiveness, and prompts sensitivity to her pain, suffering, prospects, and wishes.[45]

For Zaner, the awesome vulnerability of a patient like Mrs. Oland or, in my story, a patient like Ceci, is what "awakens the responsibility *never to take advantage of* the one who is sick or debilitated."[46]

Zaner's evocation "contra Gyges" requires a displacement of the priority of the self, a movement away from self-interest.

> There is in the embodied experience a visceral thing; to be *mindful* of this woman within her actual, concrete circumstances and compelling vulnerability. To be mindful, moreover, augers a sort of de-centering, an elemental ec-stasis as it pulls me *beyond* myself *to* her, vigilant to *her*. What and who she is, what and who I am, she and I, that odd pronominal 'self' each of us shelters, nourishes, conceals or, infrequently, reveals – are in no way given at the beginning of each life. "Self" is not something which everyone acquires at birth, whole and entire."[47]

The idea of the self who emerges from that very responsibility and freedome to share in the vulnerability of the Other nods to Spiegelberg's assertion that being thrown into existence obligates us to Others equally subjected to such an affront to our freedom. Zaner's idea of *self as responsible* also points to the relational dynamic of responsibility – it is *in response* to another, in the concrete, discrete circumstances and specific encounter, the transcendent connection in the mundane encounter – that *one becomes* a responsible self. Without the freedom to choose to respond, there is no responsibility in *my* response.

Zaner talks about Ms. Oland's situation as exemplifying "a Socratic dialogue, with its characteristic *a-poria* – that essential moment in which an interlocuter feels set upon, overcome by not knowing and by an equally strong sense of having to know."[48] This deep need to know – experienced and witnessed as vulnerability – emerges in the questions and openness that become the possibility for dialogue, for discovering meaning. Zaner writes,

> To question is to open oneself up to (or find oneself opened up by), to acknowledge a vital not-knowing and need to know – thus it is to stand ready to listen and to recognize whatever responsively and responsibly speaks to one's crisis … The question is an *appeal* to the *other* to share one's own questioning, ignorance, and search.[49]

For Zaner, and in my experiences, we do that through sharing stories about what got us to this moment, with these strangers, who may help us identify and work through what all matters now and next, and what meanings we might find or create. Especially given that vulnerabilities are often overlapping and interwoven, requiring more than one response, illustrating layers of responsibility as seen in reflecting back on the encounter with Ceci's family, Pastor Vera, and Dr. Boyard.

### Responsibility En Masse

In the "We Are Power" encounter, I tried to respond to the appeal for conversation, for dialogue, to the physician's and social worker's request to help to get clear about the unknowing of *what to do* in the face of Ceci's devastating "natural causes" vulnerability and her family's devastated, not-knowing vulnerability. In the group conversation, I kept attempting to invite shared exploration of and engagement with the questions at hand: what makes sense for Ceci and why? How do we know what we do, and what we still need to know? What is fitting and why? I aimed for what Zaner describes as

> a vital form of speaking and listening to and with the other is *dialogue* in its core form: in admitting and telling my not-knowing and need to know, I reveal and share who and what I am, and in this, *invite* the other to do so with me – trusting that the other will not take advantage of me in my not-knowing, my vulnerability.[50]

I invited Pastor Vera and Dr. Boyard to speak, to share what they understood as fitting for Ceci in the hopes they could hear each other's need, representing Ceci's needs. Yet their distinct understandings of Ceci's vulnerability demanded action from the other, and at the same time, claimed the power to write the story of this encounter, to tell what happened and how *they knew* what to do for Ceci.

In Hoffmaster, Spiegelberg, and Zaner – and in my own experiences – the challenge of how to respond and where to focus responsibility is sharp when multiple vulnerabilities are experienced and revealed. In the "We Are Power" experience, I could only recognize and respond to the deep connection between experiences of vulnerability and responsibility in the dialogue with an intentional, aimed-for openness. However, when that opening cracked wider than expected, we each were made vulnerable and rendered responsible by and for *each* other. Pastor Vera, standing in the place of, as the face, of Ceci's deep vulnerability actually highlighted Dr. Boyard's vulnerability – and mine, as the ethics consultant. She demanded care of *this person* – not just the standard of care for *a patient* – and Dr. Boyard responded, which highlighted her sense of responsibility – just as her sudden exit revealed her vulnerability. Pastor Vera's demand for Ceci's care disrupted the routine of Dr. Boyard's mundane, taken-for-granted decision-making role, and stripped away the armor of her role as a physician. She was exposed and revealed by her very human response in our later conversation: she was angry, scared, vulnerable. In the presence of her vulnerability, I felt compelled and drawn to hold a similar space open for dialogue with her as I had tried to do with Ceci's family and with Dr. Boyard in the earlier meeting. In Boyard's office, I think I managed to hold open space in that quiet listening and pause for reflection on Ceci's dying, yet I was left vulnerable in my very engagement: standing (or sitting, in that exact moment) in solidarity with the shaken.[51] I was overwhelmed, in those moments, wondering what to make of it all, how to understand it all, and not knowing what comes next – in my responses and responsibility to these fellow existers, or for myself and my practice.

Looking back, I can see how I struggled in those moments, to understand, make sense of, or find meaning in the shifting movements of that encounter – from recognitions of collective vulnerability, from not-knowing and uncertainty to the varied appeals to power and authority, to the vulnerability revealed in Dr. Boyard's unexpected response and the shift within the family to their own sense of religious or spiritual power in response to their own and Ceci's vulnerability. There were no clear lines of argument or analysis, no clear answers – even the needs and demands were jumbled together in conflicting cacophony of the ongoing, evolving question: how was I to respond, and to whom, in order to be responsible?

This is, perhaps, the sharpest kind of vulnerability I encountered and still carry – which I still *re-experience* in recollecting these interactions – and still experience when I encounter them anew – as I often do. Thinking about ongoing experiences of uncertainty, of questioning my responsibility in this encounter, and in all those before and after, I find myself returning to Zaner's astute observation that "even an authentic need does not itself guarantee a relevant response."[52] Though in Zaner's, story, the potential gap between need and response is specifically in the context of a patient and her husband, the same kind of uncertainty about the engagement with the dialogue is present for everyone involved – including the ethics consultant. The same uncertainty and potential gap stands out in my reflections on my encounter with Ceci's family and care team. I asked questions in hope and trust my questions would be heard and engaged by the others with a seriousness similar to the kind that motivated my need to know and unknowing – because mine was generated by the need-to know and not knowing of these very others. I tried to create and hold open dialogue that could recognize and respond to the various vulnerabilities prowling the room. However, as Zaner points out and I experienced fully, "The issue which dialogue must confront, then, is not so much that of the character of the questioner, but that of the one addressed by the questioner, the listener and responder."[53] They had to discern and trust my character and anticipate my response – and I had to do the same for them. Asking questions – especially ones that reveal and expose what is most at stake, what is our deepest need – is to embody and to face vulnerability. In doing so, even the act of asking demands care and "forbids manipulation or violence."[54] Zaner continues,

> the dialogic act is thus centered on a dialectic between vulnerability and power, and harbors both an immense hope and a profound risk: hope that some form of help – whether cure or only comfort – will be at hand. Risk too, is that one's vulnerability may serve only as a wedge into being taken advantage of, deceived or coerced. Both hope and risk are combined ... in an act of self-disclosure, at the very moment when the self is deeply and unavoidably vulnerable.[55]

In the story of Ceci, her family and Pastor Vera, and Dr. Boyard and me, the central and decentering vulnerability of the patient – Ceci – revealed not only the power and the vulnerability of everyone involved but that our vulnerabilities and responsibilities were ongoing. Though Dr. Boyard's decision in that dialogue resolved some types of unknowing, others bloomed like a mushroom cloud, with devastation and risk, vulnerability and need, anger and confusion lingering in the air, seeping into the groundwater, being carried forward by those involved.

I found myself with the question of whether and how to continue supporting Ceci's family and found an answer in their acknowledgement of both vulnerability and power. I was left with the question of whether and how to respond to Dr. Boyard's startling reflections on her own vulnerability in my encounter with her unexpectedly exposed human vulnerability of *not* understanding, of *not* finding meaning. Zaner is again helpful here for making sense of and responding to Dr. Boyard's acute exposure and what this encounter revealed of my own. Zaner writes in his concluding paragraphs,

> There is reason to hesitate just here: to experience a vital need to understand and be understood is to undergo the experience of not knowing and thus questioning, and that is to open oneself up by telling one's vital need to others. To tell others is to invite them to share. To communicate and to assure that one will listen. The critical need-to-know is invariably passionate in its utterance. The language of the initial need is this *passion* (urgent questioning) which seeks another's *com-passion* (responses which are responsible and responsive).[56]

Even when the situation and dialogue unfolded to give direction or allow for responsive responses to some, my responsibility as the ethics consultant didn't resolve or diminish, and my questions, my unknowing, did not and have not resolved.

**Stories Are Responsibilities**

In reflecting back on my practice in this story – remembered and written here – I can see my efforts toward com-passion in opening space for dialogue: for Ceci's brother and aunties, and Pastor Vera, to make their demands, to appeal to the doctors, the hospital, to appeal to *me* to relieve their unknowing. I don't know if it helped or mattered at all. I can see my efforts toward com-passion in my sitting and listening to Dr. Boyard in her distress, her vulnerability, of feeling powerless, to her sense of failure that she didn't help Ceci in the ways *she* thought most important (by ending what she saw as Ceci's suffering). I responded to Dr. Boyard's uncertainty and need to be heard by listening, *hard.* I do not know if it helped. I do not know if it was the response she needed or thought she might need. Which means I carry my own unknowing, my own vast vulnerability with me from that encounter through all the eons since – and that I still need to learn from and understand these experiences with others.

In order for that learning to become part of our practice, we have a responsibility to share our stories: articulating our specific experiences of consultation practices as a way of learning, with others, what it is we actually do, and what matters or doesn't, what works or doesn't, and maybe even to understand what we do when we're responding to a vulnerable other (or others) asking for help.

That question of what to do – or even what not to do – in the face of vulnerability and potential for harm reverberates through clinical encounters like the one with Ceci and her family and care team. Vulnerability generates responsibility which generates other kinds of vulnerability, especially if we dare to give voice, reveal our form and our face in the process and experiences of sharing stories about these encounters. And yet, if we don't share the experience of doing the work of consultation, of being exposed to and exposing the unchosen and unavoidable vulnerabilities in a clinical encounter, of discovering responsibilities already and always greater than our abilities and intentions, we'll miss the opportunity to learn something together. Even if it is *only* the practice of how to speak with passion – and seek and receive com-passion in return.

## Notes

1  Zaner, Richard M. (2004). *Conversations on the Edge: Narratives of Ethics and Illness*. Washington, DC: Georgetown University Press. p. xii (Quoting James Agee and Walker Evans (1969). *Let Us Now Praise Famous Men*. New York, NY: Houghton Mifflin. p. 11).
2  James, William (1992). The Sentiment of Rationality. In *Writings: 1878–1899*. New York, NY: Library of America. pp. 515–518; James, William (1992). The Will to Believe. In *Writings: 1878–1899*. New York, NY: Library of America. p. 451.
3  Hoffmaster, Barry (2006). What does vulnerability mean? *Hastings Center Report* 36 (2):38–45. p 38.
4  Hoffmaster, 39–40.
5  Hoffmaster, 40.
6  *Ibid.*
7  *Ibid.*
8  *Ibid.*
9  *Ibid.*
10  Hoffmaster, 42.
11  *Ibid.* 43.
12  *Ibid.* 42.
13  *Ibid.* 44.
14  *Ibid.*
15  Spiegelberg, Herbert (1986). Ethics for Fellows in the Fate of Existence. In *Steppingstones Toward an Ethics for Fellow Existers: Essays 1944–1983*. Dordrecht: Kluwer Academic. pp. 199–218.
16  Spiegelberg, 201.
17  Zaner, Richard M. (2010). On the Telling of Stories. In Osborne P. Wiggins and Annette C. Allen (eds.), *Clinical Ethics and the Necessity of Stories: Essays in Honor of Richard M Zaner*. Cham, Switzerland: Springer. pp. 193–210.
18  Spiegelberg, 204–205.
19  *Ibid.* 203.
20  *Ibid.* 204–205.
21  *Ibid.* 204.
22  *Ibid.* 205.
23  *Ibid.* 210.
24  *Ibid.* 206.
25  *Ibid.* 207.
26  *Ibid.* 207.
27  *Ibid.* 208.
28  I would note that this is even more acute of an issue in the current era of reckoning around how many types of "luck" are contingent upon and structured by social, structural and institutional biases.
29  *Ibid.* 209.
30  *Ibid.* 210.
31  Spiegelberg, 212–213.
32  *Ibid.* 217.
33  *Ibid.* 218.
34  *Ibid.*
35  Walker, Margaret Urban (1993). Keeping moral space open new images of ethics consulting. *Hastings Center Report* 23 (2):33–40.
36  Zaner, Richard M. (2000). Power and hope in the clinical encounter: A meditation on vulnerability. *Medicine, Health Care and Philosophy* 3 (3):263–273 (hereafter "Power").
37  *Ibid.* 266
38  *Ibid.*
39  *Ibid.* 267.
40  *Ibid.* 267.
41  *Ibid.* 268.
42  Zaner uses Plato (1961). "The Republic" in Hamilton, Edith and Cairns, Huntinton (eds.), *Plato: The Collected Dialogues*. Bollingen Series LXXI. Princeton, NJ: Princeton University Press.
43  Zaner, "Power," 269.
44  *Ibid.* 270.
45  *Ibid.* 270.

46  Zaner is quoting Spiegelberg, Herbert (1975). Good fortune obligates: Albert Schweitzer's second ethical principle. *Ethics* 85:227–234. p. 232.
47  *Ibid.* 270.
48  *Ibid.* 271.
49  *Ibid.* 271.
50  *Ibid.* 271.
51  Patočka, Jan. (1996). *Heretical Essays in the Philosophy of History* (E. Kohák, Eds., J. Dodd, Trans.). Chicago, IL: Open Court. p. 134.
52  Zaner, "Power," 272.
53  *Ibid.*
54  *Ibid.*
55  *Ibid.*
56  *Ibid.* 274.

## Bibliography

Agee, James and Evans, Walker (1969). *Let Us Now Praise Famous Men*. New York, NY: Houghton Mifflin.

Hoffmaster, Barry (2006). What does vulnerability mean? *Hastings Center Report* 36 (2):38–45.

James, William. (1992) The Sentiment of Rationality. In *Writings: 1878–1899*. New York, NY: Library of America. pp. 504–539.

James, William. (1992). The Will to Believe. In *Writings: 1878–1899*. New York, NY: Library of America. pp. 457–479.

Patočka, Jan. (1996). *Heretical Essays in the Philosophy of History* (E. Kohák, Eds., J. Dodd, Trans.). Chicago, IL: Open Court.

Plato (1961). The Republic. In Hamilton, Edith and Cairns, Huntington (eds.), *Plato: the Collected Dialogues*. Bollingen Series LXXI. Princeton, NJ: Princeton University Press.

Spiegelberg, Herbert (1975). Good fortune obligates: Albert Schweitzer's second ethical principle. Ethics 85:227–234.

Spiegelberg, Herbert (1986). Ethics for Fellows in the Fate of Existence. In Steppingstones Toward an Ethics for Fellow Existers: Essays 1944–1983. Dordrecht: Kluwer Academic. pp. 199–218.

Walker, Margaret Urban (1993). Keeping moral space open new images of ethics consulting. *Hastings Center Report* 23 (2):33–40.

Zaner, Richard M. (2000). Power and hope in the clinical encounter: A meditation on vulnerability. *Medicine, Health Care and Philosophy* 3 (3):263–273.

Zaner, Richard M. (2004). *Conversations on the Edge: Narratives of Ethics and Illness*. Washington, DC: Georgetown University Press. p. xii.

Zaner, Richard M. (2010). On the Telling of Stories. In Osborne P. Wiggins and Annette C. Allen (eds.), Clinical Ethics and the Necessity of Stories: Essays in Honor of Richard M Zaner. Cham, Switzerland: Springer. pp. 193–210.

# 6 Clinical Storytelling and Fragments of Experiences

*Part I: Acknowledgement:* **It Is Impossible to Speak … and Monstrous Not to Mention**

*Later That Same Day: The "Cameron Story"*

I don't have any words. None adequate – what feels like none left – despite the fact that I can feel them building, bubbling, pressured from the cauldron of the day's experiences. But none of them are enough – and I know this going in. I know this before I begin. I don't really know why I begin – what the point is – and who would believe me if I started. Or what I imagine they would do or could do – especially if I never stopped. I wonder if I could ever stop once I started, if I were to start. Which may be why I try to frame and limit and caveat and qualify whatever comes out – as a way of trying to contain the words that cannot, are unable to express the experience.

So I begin, to try with words to transmit the rapidly rising heartbeat that was suddenly behind my ear instead of unnoticed, underneath my chest wall where it belongs. To convey how I got distracted by the sheen of sweat that climbed, clammy as a slug's trail up my neck and across my face, liquifying the too-expensive anti-aging serum I've started applying each morning, a secular ritual of self-care, rendered meaningless and garishly frivolous as I met the eyes of the dying woman, three years my junior. Her wasted legs stuck out from under the hospital blanket, no thicker than my matronly arms and I wanted to pat her stork-thin ankle softly as she writhed, tensely, but I'd only met her and, for her, my presence was supposed to be therapeutic in its institutional, not interpersonal, role. Instead of reaching out to touch her, the calming contact my body craved to offer and that might have dispelled some of the energy of what I felt of that therapeutic need – hers and mine – I fell back on conventions and role. And all that energy, pent up and building, turned inward and burned me out, under skin to outer layers.

I didn't faint. Although when the others' voices took six steps back through an unseen tunnel and the hazy film descended without warning, I looked down as if collapse was coming. I wondered if my awareness of it could be enough to stave off a loss of consciousness, but I felt my tongue thicken before I knew I needed to speak. I turned away in the middle of Cameron's story, with her tears about pain and fighting for so long, and I leaned back toward the door while she said she was afraid of dying and that she needed to have something of good news, even if only here at the end.

I heard her finish that thought as I turned to the hospice nurse, between me and the nearest exit, and something resembling, "sorry … need …" worked its way through my teeth. Her nursing instincts kicked in, and one hand on each elbow, arm around my back, she propelled and supported me through the doorframe: chattering in the soothing voice nurses use to knit calm from the

DOI: 10.4324/9781003354864-12

swirling threads of confusion, fear, and embarrassment that attend malfunctioning bodies. She got me to a chair at the nurses' station right outside and asked the bedside nurse to bring water. The part of me trained for clinical observations marveled through my haze at their graceful choreography: reading the situation in a moment, the bedside nurse brought the water, graham crackers, and a cool, wet washcloth as well.

I laughed at myself, of course, as my shaking hands tried to unbutton my shirt cuffs. And when the patient's partner came out, away from her dying love to check on the woman who was supposed to be helping to take care of them, my blush deepened and my apologies staccatoed out. I demurred from her suggestion that I needed to get my feet up and my head down, even while she told me she was an emergency medicine technician. I responded with thanks – recognizing through the fuzz of my slowly re-orienting faculties that she was needing to care for something fixable, treatable, recoverable. Halfway through my demurral, I realized I could have helped her (and myself) by saying yes, could have helped those around me by letting them help me. My pride, my embarrassed and collapsed commitments to some idea of professionalism reared up and images of getting back in the saddle, up on the bike, nose to the grindstone, strapping the skis back on buffeted me alongside my sense of "I'm a professional, dammit!" As if professional meant unfeeling, disembodied, unaffected. As if all those metaphors, thrown around as lauding character and resilience, don't really invoke re-inserting one's soft body into a context of urgency, danger, and uncertainty from which one was just ejected, whether by happenstance or choice or necessity. I thanked her, and lied that I was fine, and promised I would rejoin them in a moment. She nodded, then patted my shoulder. The hospice nurse opened the door and followed the kind woman back to her love, dying just out of sight.

I sipped my water bottle, patted my face with the washcloth I had re-soaked with the dregs, pressing it into my eyelids, grateful my middle-aged vanity hadn't gone so far as to include mascara. I watched the bedside nurse look at the informational website about the End-of-Life Options Act – medical aid in dying – outlining the process steps of providing a patient with a lethal dose of medicine to end their life that my department put together to provide a Frequently Asked Questions for managing just such an untenable and impossible situation as this woman's. The nurse had seemed apprehensive when I had shown him the website earlier that morning, and grateful for the information I had provided. He looked calmer than I did now: I saw him watching me out of his professional eye – probably counting my pulse from the tics of my neck veins. I supposed I appeared stable, since he didn't stop me when I got back up to re-enter the patient's room, to finish what I had started.

I moved slowly toward the door, trembling with need, and uncertain how to begin again. How to apologize for being disruptive after having just explained that part of my job was to make sure this woman was as little disrupted as possible by the institutional logistics required to fulfill her request for medical aid-in-dying, for the lethal medication that would slow her heart, stop her breathing, that she hoped would end her pain and her suffering. My shame was suffocating. This woman wanted dignity of spirit and mind while her body was failing. I couldn't even demonstrate dignity with my own body, my presence. Even though I had prepared: had read the charts and talked with key people; had cleared my head and reviewed the law; had nearly memorized our institutional process. Even though I had warmed up in talking with the bedside nurse and hospice nurse, had kept my cool in morally and even emotionally challenging moments in other consultations. I had never had such an experience in a consult, when my body gave out without notice or regard to what I needed from it. I had never fainted – or come near to fainting – ever in my life. I had not, in some time, experienced this sense of deep connection with such an anguished need and my own need to help. Here, now, those needs were met and fulfilled by the role, and yet were unmet and complicated by the interpersonal, the affiliation, the embodiment – the *human*.

As I came out of my near faint, along with my reflexive laugh I had a moment of realizing why there is such a push behind systems and algorithms and checklists and matrices in this field of clinical ethics. They allow for the distance and the distancing that institutional roles – and our discomfort with discomfort – seem to put into place. It seems easy enough to follow guidelines so that all their correct boxes have been ticked. But the algorithms and checking boxes, the protocols and even the explanation of defined steps do not take into account, are *unable* to account for looking into the aged eyes of someone three years younger than myself, asking for me to make sure she can die as she imagines peaceful dying to be. Whose naked question of "Will it hurt?" surprised an answer of "I don't know" out of me – which truth she acknowledged, even as the others rush to reassure her. I found myself qualifying my honesty with, "We've never had someone complete the process here, but the reports from Oregon and Washington State over the past 20 years ..." which allowed me and the others to retreat from her experience into the evidence, the details, even as her eyes registered the truthfulness of the unfiltered response. Or I hoped that's what I saw, and not a missed clue of overwhelming pain and existential dread and hurt from the honesty.

After my nearly falling out of the room, they welcomed me back into the conversation and dismissed my apologies with the warmth of people facing their own and a loved one's death, whose attention cannot and need not be bothered by a clinician's Big Feelings about what's going on. I found myself grateful for their graciousness in both allowing me to continue to be present and for not to calling foul and writing off the whole engagement. They took my card, we exchanged thanks, and briefly reviewed plans again before I exited, more gracefully than before, I hoped. The hospice nurse stuck by me, following me around the unit as we looked for the nurse manager to tell her about what we had learned, what the plans were. And when we couldn't find her, the hospice nurse followed me down to the plaza, waiting until I found a sit-down spot on a sunshiny bench. She said, "It's happened to me before. In really intense conversations. There's no real reason why – just sometimes it hits you when you're with them. At least you didn't fall." And she smiled as she walked away, and I stared after her, with no words.

### *Part II: Resolution:* Lessons Learned in Sharing Stories

I get stuck by the feeling of having no words, despite spilling 1,500 of them on the page about this one clinical ethics encounter. What's the point of capturing any of this – all that I've written – or trying to capture in words that can barely confirm the waves of emotion, the shifting depths of attention required, the vertigo of standing so close to the abyss of another's suffering? What is the point when it may send you teetering on, perhaps over the edge? And why write the story when writing, in some ways, reproduces, refreshes, continues the awkwardness and the agony, the uncertainty and inadequacy of the words – spoken in the moment, and written down after. Why rehash, repeat, relive, *especially* when even having such documentation puts you at risk of scrutiny, criticism, second-guessing, Monday-morning quarterbacking, from one's future self (at the very least) and with a certainty, if published or presented, from peers who will listen and tsk-tsk and what if and "Well, in *our* approach ..." All of which adds another layer, turning weighty self-reflection into distressing self-criticism – Did I fail? Was it just me? – where articulation of one's personal experiences is often dismissed as idiosyncratic (and hence irrelevant) at best, as immature and inadequate (and hence irrelevant) at its harshest.

However, there are important and often unacknowledged defects in those responses just mentioned, especially the conventional idea that there is nothing gained, nothing learned from writing down, getting it out, sharing it and airing it like one's hole-y sheets and stained shirts blowing on the clothesline. The idea and the commitment that I am pursuing here, is that in caring enough to write it and to share it, new insights can emerge – something unnoticed and incubated in the task-oriented mind, and that in writing it down, presenting it to others for engagement, even critique, there is the opportunity of learning from others, at each step of the way.

It took me years to see it. Lots of re-reading and conversation and stuttering efforts to make sense among the potential meanings. I see it, though. The lesson of the "Cameron story," as I call it, is that the story isn't about Cameron, as the particular patient. Nor is the lesson about Cameron as a type of patient. Or about Cameron at all, in some ways. It's not about End-of-Life Option Act and medical aid in dying. Or clinical training. Or the resilience and steadfastness we expect of ourselves (how could *I faint*?). It's not even really about the role of the clinical ethics consultant – although that was one of the domains of inquiry I engaged during the process of writing about this experience and trying to tell this story. All of these themes and ideas and topics are areas available for probing and questioning in the "Cameron story" which is actually *my* story. But what matters for me, what this story illustrates most sharply, are the experiences and thus the real significance of telling these stories and the challenges of doing so.

We don't often talk about or share our experiences of what it is like to try to share our experiences, or about storytelling as a process of learning. Over time. With others. Unfolding in fragments. We don't talk about the process of getting out of our experiences and sharing them as *our* stories, which Wolff notes is part of the wonder of surrender-and-catch – that we *can* get out of our experiences sometimes:

> As soon as out of our crisis, we are able to talk, we have taken the first step towards transcending it … This very conviction, that talking about it may lead to its transcendence clearly distances us aloft from the crisis: it makes a beginning toward defining it – as one that can be transcended by relevant speech, that is speech entailing right action. The person who can speak about his crisis is no longer in an "extreme situation." For he has asserted his reason and his freedom, the autonomy given to man and within its limits, he knows what he must do and what not.[1]

The hope that we can possibly learn from a crisis, or extreme situation, and understand something in it is a radical hope. And yet, to get out of an experience sometimes requires going even deeper into understanding it, as was the case with my "Cameron story." Going deeper into the story is a way to understand more clearly what actually mattered, and whether such meanings can be learned, then possibly explained.

I wrote the "Cameron story" after I told it. I told it after I'd lived it. And then after I wrote it, I told it again. And then wrote about it again. And this was just in the first week.

From listening and telling *in the clinical encounter*, I found myself telling and listening with Stuart, my boss/friend/teacher, sitting in his office, my hands shaking and my breath ragged as I cried my shame and worry about failure and harming those I'd meant to help. Stuart encouraged me to write down, to capture the experience before it got altered in time or by further reflection. Recollection – the activity of remembering and rethinking the encounter – was crucial to the fact that I wrote it at all rather than letting it get washed over and away by the waves of next consult and the next.[2]

I scrawled the "Cameron story" down in one fell swoop but then it sat there, looking back at me, and I've been trying ever since to figure out what to do with it, how to share it, whether to share it, what it represents or how I can learn from it, whether others might be able to as well. As Sven Barker wrote in *The Art of Time in the Memoir*,

> I have come to recognize that memory is an irrational, even counter-intuitive ecologist: obeying the most obscure private laws and raising arcs of the central questions facing the memoirist. What are the terms of mattering; what was actually important?[3]

In writing and sharing it, the "Cameron story" became about more than the "events" of that experience. The struggle for me has been discovering what matters, what was actually important such that it needs to be shared.

The "Cameron story" is both mine to share and becomes something else in the sharing. In trying to write and tell the story of this encounter, the moment expanded, like musician Joe Henry says a song does, letting us become buoyant in the moment, where more becomes available to and through those listening than was available to the initial storyteller.[4] After all, no one else will have *that* particular experience of nearly fainting in a patient's room – but others might have an experience where their clinical moment becomes a story – one where listening and telling and writing and sharing that story becomes its own moral encounter – with self and others.

As part of the practice of learning about and thinking about practice from and in conversation with others, Stuart also invited me to tell and listen as part of our CECS Case Review, scheduled serendipitously for the following Monday. And so, I did. I gave the account – I told the clinical story out loud with colleagues and peers, who were also friends and supporters. Their questions and probing let me go further into the experience than I had before, even in the experience, and helped me to discover and get more out of the experience than my own allowed.

It circles back around – eventually, and yet, the moments of recognition always surprise me.

### *My Story – Clinical Ethics Consultation Service Case Review*

It was a different table this time – with different people. Samantha, Andy, Ken, and Stuart from my professional environment blurring with Mindy, Dan, Jan, Mark, and Kyle from my clinical training days. But, somehow, it seemed like it was the same moment. It had requisite essentials: deeply attentive, concerned and curious, open and thoughtful peers who were listening and talking. Colleagues thinking with me about a moment when the mundane unfurled into surrender thrown by a connection, an affiliation with the moral weight perceived in another's suffering. The questions were the same: lively and urgent, trying to understand what "ethics" meant and what it means to "do ethics consultation" in the experience of disruption.

Stuart asked what made this moment different from any other consultation? What had I learned about the practice, the roles of Clinical Ethics consultation? I went back and forth: personal and professional, embodied and experiential: philosophical in the deepest sense of rigorous inquiry. I struggled to explain what it was like to be in that moment, overwhelmed by responsibility – and feeling like I was failing at it, even in the actual moments which gave evidence that I was fulfilling it.

It was no different from any other encounter and yet it was so different from every other. It was a moment when the preparation, orientation, discipline, and attention – the careful attention and attunement – *worked*. I encountered, witnessed the full rawness of anguish and fear, bravery and sorrow, this woman's desperate attempts to manage and control – through access to medical aid-in-dying– the uncertainty and unfolding in her dying. That rawness transcended my desperate and careful attempts to manage and control this uncertain and unfolding process with her. The links between the therapeutic and the administrative, the professional and the personal, the process and the outcome all commingled into each other in an engagement that exceeded requestor, request, and respondent.

Around that conference table, days later, it was in talking through and probing, with my colleagues, that bits and pieces of the encounter became clearer. The demands of a description, for an accurate accounting, of telling a story, brought forward the moments of self-reflection on even the most mundane instinctive act of reaching out to touch the dying woman's foot – that were crystalline in my hyper focus of the moment and became sharp in my remembrance and re-presentation to my colleagues. In Stuart's retrospective probing, I could see the moment of attunement was recognizing that Cameron asked for my presence through the role (the ethics person to explain the institutional process) because of her therapeutic need for reassurance and management of her anxiety and terror. I responded – had prepared to respond – with the administrative as therapeutic – to provide the information, the reassurance of process and communication. Yet in that moment of attending to that therapeutic need and responding with an administrative therapy, we were undone by our success.

Cameron surrendered to her relief by talking experientially about her fear and her dying – to the point where she collapsed in on her own tears and choked words and her gratitude for my assurance of institutional, clinical support. And I was so close to her, so attentive and open and attuned to discovering what was going on, that I surrendered, undone and disrupted, to her expression of relief, to her collapse into the moment. My surrender, backwards down the growing tunnel of a vasovagal loss of consciousness, was no less disruptive for its silence. Our affiliation in that moment was both therapeutic and held glimpses of potential harms – to each of us. Her surrender brought forth a catch of recognitions, which opened into my own surrender.

So, back to Stuart's question: What Did I Learn? What's the "catch"? The catch is that such wild and total involvement was unavoidably unpredictable. Perhaps my biggest challenge – my error, if you will – was approaching with the idea that my responsibility was predetermined by the role of ethics consultant, contained by what had been asked for in this request: an administrative framing. I confronted the idea – perhaps my unacknowledged wish – that my engagement could be predetermined and constrained – limited by and to what was asked, somehow able to avoid what might be discovered and demanded in the moment. That perhaps for *this one*, this time when I was most anxious and uncertain, that I would be involved only with the process, not the provision of care. Because the idea of caring for someone who was in the fully embodied injustice of agonized dying was terrifying. Perhaps even deeper, I held some hope that if I was so distanced, so predetermined, I would be protected from whatever such demands might be – including the feared recognition that I might *not* be able to meet them.

In some mix of the reasons Stuart rattled off as suggestions as to why I was so disrupted or what made this different (e.g., our age similarity; the administrative responsibilities, that it was about aid-in-dying; that it was a Monday; personal stress, etc.) I recognized that I had gotten caught by thinking of the encounter with Cameron was different because of the bureaucratic requirements around aid-in-dying. And so, instead of approaching with my usual strategies and attention and orientation toward discovery, I went in *assuming a role*, relying on what I *knew* and could explain to fulfill a role, no more, no less. Thus, I was somehow surprised and undone by the embodied experience of two simple facts that I *have* learned over the years *are* routine and regular for any and every consultation. First, that the engagement in a consultation exceeds what is requested; and second, discovering what all matters requires alert and careful attention in the moment, followed by equally careful reflection after the encounter. I was surprised, somehow, in the moment with Cameron, to discover the fully embodied reminders that the role does not offer armor and protection, but rather puts one on the perilous, unsteady ground of moral disruption.

I also remembered, in the experience of retelling, that the moral disruption exceeds the encounter – in the moment and after. Even days later, with my vasovagal responses well-monitored and more regulated, my tears still interrupted at times during the conversation around the shiny dark conference room table. Stuart and I talked through the occasional choked-back sob and my words getting caught by a ragged sniffle. He and I were well-practiced at this point, although my distress provoked looks of concern from Samantha and Ken, and mild curiosity from Andy. Both Stuart and I pressed on, acknowledging and moving through the embodied response to the deep experience I was trying to recount and re-present. With his questions, and Samantha's, the back-and-forth volleys of storytelling examples from Andy to Samantha and back to me, and Ken's reflections on touching the stranger (from his view as a physician of the old school), my experience became clearer, richer, deeper. It became part of a different moral experience.

In the expansion of the clinical moments into reflective conversation, the recognition broke through again: that it all circles around. That preparation is insufficient for any given encounter – no matter how necessary. That each consultation, each moment is practice for the next, which will be unique and will come to serve as practice for the next. That the understanding and learning are incomplete – no matter how final the moment when an experience ends. That the responsibility is an ongoing activity – of just such engagement, of just such learning – not an achievement to be mastered or laurels to rest upon. The story isn't finished just because I left the room, or even after I have remembered and recounted the encounter. The story isn't done just because I put my pen down.

## Part III: Pursuance: Reflectively Unphilosophical Fragments or, 10 Things for Readers to Know

### First: This Is the Hardest Story I've Ever Written

This is the hardest story in the sense of being one of the most challenging clinical moments in nearly 20 years and over 1,700 consults. It is the hardest in the sense of writing it down – the moment and its hardness – knowing from the first thought about making the first effort, that the writing would be inadequate, would be *insufficient* to do justice to or capture the moment, the moral engagement, the human connections in clinical ethics work. Yet I found myself compelled to do so anyway, to try to speak it, name it, write it, share it. It is the sternest story, too, because of what it reveals about clinical ethics work at its core: that it always carries with it the possibility that we are "searching in a dark cellar at midnight for a black cat that isn't there"[5] – believing there is a meaning or a sense that can be made among us if we work together, if we try and trust, and care enough. It means being willing to go forward, in what Zaner describes as freedom,[6] knowing that despite our training, practice, skills, good intentions, and institutional authority: we may not be able to help in any given moment – may not be able to hold the space for those in need to catch their breath and make sense of whatever impossible circumstance they find themselves in at a given moment. It means acknowledging we are now a part of that impossible circumstance with them, and so we may need others to help us catch our breath, too.

The impossible circumstances of clinical ethics encounters remind of a children's book my youngest daughter received, Cori Doerrfeld's *The Rabbit Listened*, where a child's elaborate castle of building blocks is unexpectedly destroyed by a random flock of birds.[7] A parade of animals come to suggest ways the child could respond, or with offers to "fix" things. The chicken offered to talk talk talk, the elephant suggested yelling, the ostrich recommended burying one's head in the sand, while the snake offered to help knock over someone else's blocks. None of the proffered fixes helped, and the child remained in distress and uncertainty about what to do. The book pivots with the arrival of the rabbit, who simply comes to sit with the child. Eventually the child begins to talk.

And rage. And cry. And fantasize about lashing out. And as the rabbit listens, the child begins to imagine what comes next, to dream forward – not to recreate what was lost, but to build from the pieces of what was left. The listening, the presence, the space created by the listening helped the child identify, articulate, and move forward into a future of activity and choices that fit with their experiences, what Richard Zaner would call the "aftermaths" of the encounter. The child could tell a new story, with someone who listened.

### Second: Meaning-Making in Clinical Encounters Is Not an Epistemic Project – It Is a Moral Activity Requiring Preparation and Practice

Listening and telling – as a clinical practice – elicits the stories of those in the unchosen upending of their lives by illness, injury, and the fear of death and disability, by pain and confusion and deeply uncertain futures. The sense of what is *fitting* for a given clinical ethics encounter, that is, the most significant meanings, are not found, lurking on their own, to be ferreted out by the clarity of our policies or processes, nor can these be brought in and applied from the search beams of books and theories without overwhelming those who have been adjusting to the fugitive character of their suddenly strange and different lives. Clinical storytelling is both necessary and insufficient, even when framed by its own terms and traditions, its own rhythms of call and response and meaning making. And this is why clinical storytelling – accounting for our experiences – is both the most natural thing in the world to do and also a deeply weird thing to articulate. If taken seriously, we have to begin with the acceptance that the storytelling – the clinical accounting – for others' stories as patients, families, clinicians and for ours as ethics consultants – already falls short of its need and promise before it even begins, no matter how much education, training, and preparation we bring to our practice.

For clinical storytelling as a moral activity, being prepared means bringing previous experience to each *sui generis* moment, each new encounter. It means we have to midwife the experiences that are emerging, and get to help birth-catch the bloody squirming story: wiping free and soothing the raw embodiment, helping clear its throat so it can scream and sing into the human chorus for a moment. Part of the work is helping to coach the person breathing in gasps, as they try to get out all that matters, all that has been growing, meanings that they have nurtured and held close under their heart, perhaps without knowing it.

Listening and telling is what we do to make sense of the stories we receive. But we must do this with our own stories as well if we are to get clearer on the edges and find the hidden gems and the points of light and new songs. Aiming for such clarity requires that these stories be about us– and we're not so good at those. We hide in them – saving the blood and guts, pathos, the harrowing moments, to explain what the patients are going through – or what clinicians face in the moments of near catastrophic physical/emotional/existential uncertainty. And the terrible secret is if we are there with them – in our role, even with all the protections of preparation and trappings of training and iron armor of institutional authority – we, too, are in it, *and we may not get out of it either.* There is no preparation that guarantees anything but possibility.

The moral moment will not be televised.

### Third: The Arc of This Chapter Is Learning to Tell My Own Story – As a Clinically and Philosophically Relevant Aspect of Practice

We are not the all-seeing eye of our own experience and as John Hardwig notes, we may be the least trustworthy narrators of what "really" happened.[8] This experience gutted me – as much in the telling of it as in the embodied moments the telling reveals. This story has gutted me in each of the myriad ways I've tried to explain its importance, its resonance since that moment, and I've struggled with *why?* Because what matters, the meaning, is not static. *E pur si muove.* Which is the reason we share with others what we do and why. We need conversation partners, interlocutors who can push us on the details, help us recall the sense and feel and sound and smell and tone – and who can invite us to go deeper into bringing our story to life, to find more in the telling than we may perceive in the moment, or later even in our own reflections.

In telling our stories to and with others, it is possible to focus on *our experiences* as clinical ethics consultants – including the hardness, the shaking, and shuddering that comes with caring and love and being human and being responsible. The intersubjective weight and connection are harder to talk about, but no less vital than the details of the consultation "questions" that we can hold at a distance, clad in the armor of our education, training, and expertise about such topics. The connections among people instantiates these as intersubjective, moral encounters and require at least a recognition that as the ethics consultants, we are involved, we care about what happens, and hence we are subject to question as much as any other participant. As Zaner writes,

> that involvement, in a word, harbors a critical question for anyone in ethics: what exactly, if anything, is the 'ethics' of 'ethics consultation'? What justifies this act, my own decision to become 'involved' in all the ways consultants invariably display?[9]

If and when we are involved, we are involved as our individual selves (even if part of a team). We aren't standing in as A Reasonable Ethicist – we are there as ourselves – with all the idiosyncratic variability and weighted responsibility that entails.

This is my story, not the story of the patient, or even her family. It is partial, particular, and deeply perspectival. This is not a polyphonic case.[10] It is kaleidoscopic and personal – which is what makes it accessible to others: as Wolfe wrote, "in surrender we are thrown back on what we really are, which is what we share with mankind."[11] This is my story shared in the hopes of gaining clarity *in the process of* sharing and offering this story to others. After all, this story reveals much about the work of clinical ethics that goes *unspoken*, unacknowledged, and yet, inescapably, must be considered vital to the practice. As I both intimated and mentioned, in this story, I engaged with a fellow human at the limits of her experience, in her crisis of being and her deeply embodied existential terror, which found voice as an *unknowing* about steps and process for medical aid-in-dying. I encountered and found myself exposed in her extremis and disruption, such that her need to make sense of what is now and what is next became mine. In meeting her there – in my therapeutic role (educated, trained, prepared within an inch of my life, institutionally authorized), I met the limits of my own experience. My extremis was my deeply embodied *unknowing*, and uncertainty about how to make sense of that "what is now and what is next" highlighted the perceived threat of not knowing what is needed in this moment, with this dying woman. Cameron and I were together in the moment and although our experiences were individuated by our particularities and uniqueness, the exposure to and bearing witness to her suffering connected with my own – resonated, vibrated. That was the moment when we might have understood each other for just a flash, that vivid flicker of lightning – before it cracked into thunder through a sky used to rumbling.

I don't know how one does this work with fellow humans in crisis, in disruption and unknowing, without the kinds of intersubjective connection and near-constant self-reflection in practice that each of my stories about clinical encounters shows, reveals. Since I don't see as much of this kind of writing, storytelling, reflection on actual practice in the literature of our field, I'm trying to share mine, share my stories with strangers, of the encounters with strangers. I'm writing and sharing these stories about my experience out of gratitude for my continued learning from all those patients, families, clinicians who have been my teachers without any idea of the gifts they were sharing.

I'm writing it, as well, for those (including myself) who might have similar kinds of experiences with these elements of responsibility at different points – or all the points – in their practice, but especially those at the beginning. Here you go. Read your futures in my entrails – I've spilled them across the page, and I'm poking through them too – hoping for a sign, an augury to make some kind of meaning, walking the lines between living and dying. [This is the part where those who would like to dismiss California (and possibly California bioethics)[12] – as woo-woo and wacky, have even more reason to do so. Why is she talking about auguries and entrails when Serious Bioethics involves Reason and Consensus? Yikes. But it doesn't always, and aye, there's the rub … and that's a whole different set of conversations for another book, another time.]

Beginnings are never-ending in this work.

### Fourth: Storytelling Carries Obligations. So Does Listening

In Barry Lopez's fable, *Crow and Weasel*, the conversations between the title characters on their travels, and their unexpected host, Badger, emphasize the importance of giving stories their proper tellings because of the power stories have. I first encountered this story through a quotation referenced in Zaner's writings, sent by my mentor in an email. Talk about happenstance. The quotation about storytelling stuck with me, such that I bought Lopez's book, for ease of rereading, and I'm sharing the lines here, gifting them forward in this context of reflection and storytelling. Badger explains the weight and the value stories have in being shared:

> "I would ask you to remember only this one thing," said Badger. "The stories people tell have a way of taking care of them. If stories come to you, care for them. And learn to give them away when they are needed. Sometimes a person needs a story more than food to stay alive. That is why we put these stories in each other's memories. This is how people care for themselves. One day you will be good storytellers. Never forget these obligations.

> No one since Mountain Lion had spoken so directly to them of their obligations, but this time Crow and Weasel were not made uncomfortable. Each could understand what Badger was talking about, and each one knew that if his life went on, he could one day know fully what Badger meant. For now, all it means was that it was good to remember and to say well what had happened, if someone asked to hear.[13]

Taking care of stories – this careful storytelling – became an element of my practice, part of the method modeled for me since the moments of rounding and Seminar at Vanderbilt. In those places and times, beginning with my adventuring and exploring in clinical contexts, all that was asked of me was whether I could listen and learn, remember well, say well what had happened, to share with those who asked to hear. Now one thing I ask of myself in professional practice is to continue those efforts, trying to be a good storyteller.

I try to share these stories I have carried for so long and to share them as stories I would have liked to read as a student – and what I would like to read now, still, to hear from others about their practice, especially in my ongoing work. This book offers written accounts of what I learned from the oral tradition and daily modeling from my teachers, from the texts and contexts I've encountered since I first stumbled into clinical ethics. From the beginning, I had Mountain Lion laying the heavy burden of obligations, and Badger reminding me to find the music of the stories, the proper registers to share what all matters. I aim to remember and to put these stories into others' memories, as I carry those put in mine.

I recognize the responsibility for taking care – caring for – those whose stories we are given and now carry ... for those whose stories they are (including myself) ... and the obligation to offer these stories to those who need them *now* to live, including at times, ourselves and each other.

### Fifth: I'm Struck by the Multiple Activities at Work in Listening-and-Telling Stories

We receive stories: listening as stories emerge from experiences, from cultural amalgamations of experiences; from imaginations and questions (often fed by experiences).

We remember: the people, the settings, the embodied richness, the thickness of details which move encounters from moments to memories. Zaner talks about thinking through a situation once out of the moment – at a remove, in memory. Elie Wiesel writes, "If he seems strange, it is because he is possessed by a strange memory, which holds pictures and words, all kinds of pictures, all kinds of words, even those belonging to others."[14] We remember to try to make sense of what we received, as well as our involvement in the ongoing story.

We reflect on the stories: we review, revise, and reconsider, with others trying to get at what it was at stake in those moments,[15] trying to sink into understandings in shared/extraordinary discourse,[16] checking ourselves out of our confidence/ease,[17] discovering the variety of perspectives available in the retelling that had to be discovered after the encounter itself, in the unfolding polyphonic case.[18]

We retell the stories: Badger's admonishments for detail and accuracy "trying to help them, by teaching him to put the parts together in a good pattern, to speak with a pleasing rhythm, and to call on all the details of memory ..." which she notes, "make me wonder at the strangeness of the world. That strangeness, that intriguing life of another people, it is a crucial thing, I think, to know."[19] We hold onto the details and discover more in the retelling – but we don't hold everything. We don't always have access to all the details a listener might need. So Zaner talks about telling stories faithfully[20]: making it up if you can't get it perfectly right in your remembering, being careful not to put others (or yourself) in the dock, or in the stocks.

### Sixth: Clinical Storytelling Is Transformative of Story, of Teller, of Listener

Clinical work requires attention to and care for the stories we share with strangers, people, our fellows in the fate of existence. We ask for and elicit and share and co-create *stories* with each other. When we enter into conversation in a clinical encounter with patients and their loved ones, clinicians and staff, we receive *their* questions, enter into *their* experiences, listen to their stories. In the later stages and even aftermaths of our work – the remembering and reflecting and retelling – we mull over what we experienced in the receiving – what we got, what we understood, what sense we made of it at the time – what sense others may have made of it – and maybe if we see it in those same ways, or now differently in the aftermaths.

Sometimes we transform those questions and experiences into stories in the chart notes and institutional reports we generate as part of our working in healthcare settings. Sometimes we transform them into whatever philosophical frame was the root of our training or is *de rigueur* at our conference or in our journals at a particular time. Nonetheless, we need to be equally clear that although these may be necessary types of accounts that we give and create for their different purposes, they are not sufficient for the actual work that we do. Being responsible in storytelling is actually the work of receiving, remembering, reflecting, and retelling: we have to understand which one we're doing – and be deliberate in these activities. They are each trying to trace some aspect of an experience, alive in the moment and available in our ongoing learning, but they are different: we must be careful not to confuse our reflecting with receiving and recognize that re-membering is not the same as retelling. To be careful stewards of stories, our own and others, we must be deliberate in how we engage them, make sense of them, and use them to make sense of other stories and experiences, perhaps unfolding in real time.

We learn through the stories we carry, that we are gifted, that we accumulate, that we help co-create. And while there is much debate about the "ethics of" and moral justification for using other peoples' stories to frame our theorizing or public writings – I have a growing commit-ment to the practice of sharing *our stories* of our experiences and clinical encounters – about what we said, did, thought, wondered, about how we moved, or didn't, listened or spoke. We need to share our stories for what we can teach each other – not because anyone else can (or should) do the same exact thing. Our stories cannot offer a script, a blueprint, or precise recipe for practice. Nor should we break our arms patting ourselves on the back, holding ourselves up exemplary. And we should not tell our stories as penance offering our encounters as an object lesson – *Mea culpa*! Beware! Don't do as I have done! The moments that elicit clinical ethics consultation are so complex that generally neither we as consultants nor those we encounter deserve the praise of an unblemished hero or the self-flagellation of the deeply repentant. "Our choices are half chance. So are everyone else's."[21] We still can and ought to share our stories, without resort to professional-self-help, seeking absolution for our clinical missteps or valida-tion of our good work.

Thus, instead of trying to strip the moment down to a type of case or demonstrate how a par-ticular communication technique worked or didn't, telling stories about *our* experiences unfolds the moment and reveals more than we may have noticed or been aware of while surrendered to another's disruption/concerns/questions. It takes seriously the weight of the encounters and con-nections – the newness of each moment for the persons enmeshed in them.

Telling stories creates convergences with similar encounters, each enriching the other.

### Seventh: The Work of Stories Is Shared Over Time

Sharing stories, listening-and-telling, giving accounts, is part of how we model the "ethics" of clin-ical ethics for those in the moral moments with us,[22] for those whose stories we are trying to learn and learn from through those conversations. We elicit and listen, we share each other's stories, tell the stories that matter to us, trying to make sense and learning to understand what all matters in a given encounter. As folk singer Dar Williams wrote,

> *I was all out of choices but the woman of voices*
> *She turned round the corner with music around her,*
> *She gave me the language that keeps me alive, she said:*
> *"I'm so glad that you finally made it here*
> *With the things you know now, that only time could tell*
> *Looking back, seeing far, landing right where we are ...*
> *and oh, you're aging well."*[23]

In clinical ethics consultation, we operate as "the woman of voices": we ask for others' stories, we probe the roots or origins of their beliefs, believing they matter (because they do), and we ask what they use to make sense of their worlds so they can imagine forward into what's next – even in the face of unknowing – helping them to connect and engage with these encounters in their own lives/stories and those of others. We have to be able to speak to and model what it is like and what it is about – and that we are with them in the sheer, unjust uncanniness of it all.

The stories and practice of telling them as fully, accurately, faithfully as possibly – emphasizing what stands out to us and recalling more detail or nuance in response to the questions of others – this dialogical communication in the middle of the clinical encounter replicates itself in our stories of clinical moments, when we share them with colleagues and peers. It's not that one story, one example, will tell us what to do or how to do the next one, or what the right answer is for any given clinical conundrum (which is, at root, a human conundrum). Sharing stories with each other helps spread their weight and beauty, which are part of what we carry into and share with others in our consultation work, from the now to the next.

For our clinical stories to be worth their telling, to be helpful and instructive not just en-tertaining, self-promoting, or cathartic releases, these stories, instead have to raise questions, to prompt or prod the reader to wonder "What if? What would it be like? What do I imagine I would do or say or think or feel and why?" or "Wow, my experience was/is different … here's how it went down in my world." They need to connect with the work and experiences of others. Not only "Oh, here's what I use to make sense of it," but also "Here's how they make *me* think about it." Clinical storytelling is not about ASBH-certified experts said "x" or this text said "y" and "Now we have consensus about how to resolve this" or "We know what not to do next time." Stories become static, even sterile, if they attempt to offer an authoritative, final word on a skill or practice element, topic or question, an ideal outcome. An example:when asked in an interview whether it was ok that as the songwriter, he doesn't know what a song is about, Joe Henry responded, "Yes! As soon as I decide, as a song is about, what it means, that's all it can ever mean. But I don't think a song serves us when it's nailed to the floor. If I think I know where a song is going, then I've kind of painted myself into a corner."[24] Our stories are not unlike songs in their shared creation of meaning: the stories we tell each other *about ourselves and our practice* fall short of their possibility if they fall into the triumphant "Mission accom-plished!"; *and* they fail if they fall into the self-flagellation of "alas if only …" Those responses allow us and our readers/peers, both, off the hook too easily, and let us avoid the persistent questions about actual practice.

In the complexity of clinical stories, we have to ask: can we actually offer our stories with the kind of openness and vulnerability and authenticity (we claim) we want from the people with whom we consult? Can we engage the questions of experience and engagement for ourselves, as phrased by Henry in the same interview mentioned above: "How do we live robustly when we know we're not always going to? How do we bring ourselves to compassion and presence when it's not always our impulse to be there?"[25]

So, the question of method that stories raise for each of us in our practice is this: Can we take seriously the questions of *how* and *what is it like* to do this work without assuming that it has all been done and it has all been worked out already?

### Eighth: Stories We Share Are Also NOT SAFE

There's an existential vulnerability inherent in exposing and offering your experiences for public review. They can reveal Dar Williams's reminder, from another song, that we "don't like to make our passions other peoples' concerns."[26] Telling our own stories is rarely safe – they can rip us wide open, turn us inside out – and publicly.

In that context, sharing stories and reflections reveals an extensive cluster of vulnerabilities: the possibility of discovering just how strange my perspective is – or just how typical and acclimated those perspectives are, as well as the possibility of revealing more to others than *we* recognize about ourselves. The writing extends beyond anything I intend it to be, it reveals and exposes more than I intend it to expose. After all, while the experiences exceed the writing   always   the writing creates its own excess of experience – always.

So why do this? Why write? What is the good in offering a partial, limited, and temporally contained, bias-laden account of an unrepeatable experience? What is the point of revealing oneself in that effort?

The point is that we might also find out that others share a similar experience, and that we might learn something from each other's particularity. As Sven Birkerts writes in *The Art of Time in Memoir:*

> The job of memoirist to give the reader both the unprocessed feeling of the world as I saw it then *and* a reflective vantage point that incorporates or suggests that those events made a different kind of sense over time. *This is the transfiguration that if done well, absolves the memoirist's reflections from the charge of self-involved navel gazing.* What makes the difference is not only the fact of the self-reflective awareness but the conversion of private into public by way of a narrative compelling the interest and engagement of the reader. The act of storytelling – even if the story is an account of psychological self-realization – is by its very nature an attempt at universalizing the specific; it assumes that there is a shared ground between teller and audience.[27]

Clinical storytelling is, at its root, the assumption, the hope even, that there *is* a shared ground between and among us, and that we can help each other understand what matters and what is meaningful in our interactions.

### Ninth: The Storytelling Reveals that We Can't Always Account for What We Do and Why

The idea of telling stories, writing about what matters and what is meaningful in our clinical interactions raises another concern and question. How do we account for (let alone write about) those momentous circumstances in situations, even moments, when we take responsibility, but that we *don't* talk about; that we *don't* account for in the typical case reports, chart notes, professional papers and presentations? Where and how do we talk about the limits of our own accounts? Because even in telling the most nuanced and detailed rendition of our experiences, we reveal that there are moments that we don't, *or won't* describe, in the encounter, or even after, in our professional accounts about the clinical encounters.

For example, there are moments in clinical ethics encounters where we know that because of what we do or don't do, what we say or don't say, someone is going to die … or is going to go on living, bound to a life of medical machines and ongoing debilitation. We know that circumstances, and things in them, change because of our involvement, in part due to whether we do or say something in this way, or in that way … We know that when the conversation is going one way, or could go another, and we see which way it might happen, and we can see the struggle of people trying to decide – we can make a decision about how the conversation will unfold because we let it happen; we make these judgments along the way. The point is that we don't articulate this as a judgment, as something for which we are responsible. At most, we may acknowledge when we make an intentional nudge. We rarely talk about the responsibility we embody and take on in these instances of others' responsibility and freedom.[28]

In my stories, Cameron would access the means to end her life and I am part of that. Ceci's family would have a different experience with her death and their grief because of my actions or inactions. So would Dr. Boyard. Whichever choices I make in an adventure as it unfolds may be ones I understand and can articulate, or I may find that there are indications that were not evident at first, or I may even discover that I am hidden by some other elements that make me obscure to myself. These recognitions, and the judgments they evoke, are a deeply moral part of clinical ethics work that we don't talk about in professional contexts, but which our storytelling might reveal –including our lack of understanding, our unknowing, and our responsibility for that unknowing.

Maybe, we don't include these in the discourse because it's better not to articulate it, not to bring this unknowing and responsibility into language so directly and explicitly. After all, if you live and work in an environment that is procedural – how would you explain the difference to your peers? Colleagues? Superiors? How do you articulate the discernment? The determination between one judgment over another? Is it possible to find time and space to speak about *your* discernment, *your* judgment – to speak about the recognition that it could always be otherwise, in a world that seeks certainty and finality, that seeks closure and teleology? Do we practice in silence, keeping these recognitions to ourselves, shielding ourselves and others from the fact that, among the recognizable possibilities, your involvement had some influence such that things turned out like they did, and you may not be sure how or why? Writing about and sharing such moments risks exposure to misinterpretation and misunderstanding. On the other hand, equally unnerving is that others might actually understand what those moments are like: they might understand us.

So then, even more sharply: why write? Why risk understanding in efforts that only expose accounts of the unconditional uniqueness, the variability, the attentiveness, *the responsibility* for those engagements when what is actually shown illustrates how little understanding there is? Why bother to invite conversation about such experiences, for which we can't even access, let alone explain, all of the assumptions, biases, and commitments we bring to our judgment, activities, and reflections? After all, it is possible to engage in this work in an instrumental way, rooted in notions of efficiency, trading on the presumptions of competence and the warrant of credentials over accounting for practice. The move toward professionalization establishes structures and procedures for efficiency, quality metrics and measurement. These structures and processes trade on just such ideas and ideals of values, of consideration and investigation of what is worthwhile – of the things that clinical ethics has claimed as its domain for a long time.

However, those same structures and procedures of professionalization – certification, in particular – resist any efforts to actually embody, engage, exemplify those value-laden activities. In philosophical traditions there is the expectation and reliance that others will probe with you, will push on assumptions and seek clarity, and maybe even understanding, as a means of living in and living through particular questions.[29] And yet, especially in instrumental or efficiency-based systems, there are whole sets of actions, of interactions, that occur in a kind of silence – of being non-calculable. There are actions taken, or not taken, for which there is then no account. In such systems – whether healthcare or academic or both – you can't always tell what's being done or not, let alone tell how it's going … and so there's an experience of constant unknowing: the house of cards may not hold up to a vigorous wind, or even the curious poking around with a penlight. Whether in an academic structure through seminars and courses or clinical cases through a systematic-model structure, clinical ethics work trades on the cachet of understanding and values and identifying and respecting what is at stake. However, the structure neither guarantees that such values will be uncovered nor that they will be respected nor responded to once identified.[30]

So how is it possible to articulate such unknowing, such uncertainty – to oneself, let alone to others, in an environment, or a field, committed to the surety of expertise and authority?

### Tenth: Storytelling Is Intersubjective and Rigorous Is Ways We May Not Appreciate

Audre Lorde, writer, womanist, philosopher, and civil rights activist, once wrote,

> It isn't that to have an honorable relationship with you, I have to understand everything, or tell you everything at once, or that I can know, beforehand, everything I need to tell you.
>
> It means that most of the time I am eager, longing for the possibility of telling you. That these possibilities may seem frightening, but not destructive, to me. That I feel strong enough to hear your tentative and groping words. That we both know we are trying, all the time, to extend the possibilities of truth between us. [31]

We have to tell stories while knowing – and resisting – our instinct to excuse ourselves, our impulse to put ourselves in the best light possible, to reconfigure the narrative to fit our preferred self-understandings. John Hardwig observed this phenomenon with humor and sharp critique – that we tell different kinds of lies in our stories, especially in our "autobiographical" stories, and that perhaps rather than rely on our own selves for an "authentic" or "real" version, we find the truth about ourselves, the meaning of a story, perhaps, in the telling and listening, in the movement between and among those sharing the dialogue.

If this is so, and my experience has been that it is certainly so, then we cannot simply tell our stories to ourselves, or write them as if no one would hear them or read them. We have to "know we are trying, all the time, to extend the possibilities of truth between us.". We have to learn the stories in the moments *and* in the telling, like Weasel and Crow in Lopez's fable, taking stories back to their people, sharing their peoples' stories with the strangers they meet along their journey. When we share stories, our listeners have the possibility – indeed, the responsibility – to push and probe and question, even challenge, our telling. Like Badger demonstrates, the questioning of others brings to light, makes clearer the nuances and details of our experience – the subtle moments of choice or response that we might gloss over in our initial presentation. We can test our ideas with and against each other. As Frolic and Ofstad make clear, our assumptions, our usual ways of seeing and being in the world become available for question when we share stories with others, even with the strangers we know the best in our communities, teams, or families.

The telling of stories – particularly the writing of stories – becomes an avenue for understanding, for making meaning of events or encounters that we may not have chosen, experiences of unknowing and uncertainty of the kind Zaner describes with Ms. Oland, structuring the moral in clinical encounters.[32] Like Finder did with the Zadeh encounter, we may scrawl down fragments of stories – compelled by the urgency and uncertainty of the encounter, just to get it out of our minds, making it available for study.[33] Yet, even in doing so, imagining no one will ever see it but ourselves (if we choose to look), we know our story exists, and we are faced with the question of whether and how and why we might share it. *That* question carries a heavy weight no matter what.

If shared, our stories may be beneficial to us, the storytellers, as well as to our listeners (or readers), and even to the other people who appear in and interact with our stories, whether as key figures or side characters. They may also be harmful to the same people. The storyteller must hold an awareness that the possibility of learning is not always beneficial, or even benign, Thus, caring for and bringing a fidelity to the story is required – for those in it, and to those listening to or reading it and for ourselves in telling. After all, if we don't share our stories, the holding-in and the keeping to ourselves can have its own harms – not sharing knowledge, certainly, and also the harm to ourselves of not learning from others' questions and probing – of not being open to others' engagement.

*The Zadeh Project* stands as an example of the rigors of sharing – and invitation to engagement, critique, reflection with others, layered and requiring attunement and affiliation to make sense of what is presented, and the vulnerability of exposing what is raised in or by what is presented. The invitation of *the Zadeh Project* – of clinical storytelling in general – is to explore and discover the provinces of meanings where others live, work, experience the world.[34] It is to welcome the anarchy of voices and cacophony of perspectives that constellate in clinical ethics encounters.[35] *Sharing Stories with Strangers* answers that invitation by offering its own constellation of encounters and reflections on them, drawing from resources and conversation partners in *still other* domains and provinces of meaning, who illuminate and sharpen what all matters in these stories, in these encounters, not just "the answer" or preferred outcomes. Like Crow realizes, watching Badger question and probe and slow down the telling of Weasel's story: hurrying to get to "the point" or "the big picture" can easily miss the details and nuances that make a story unique, and hence understandable. Insisting that working through the details primarily to get to "the choice" shows the drive to expedite, to reduce to the highlights – or an unwillingness to see things unfold – that differentiates an "ethics case" from a story of a clinical encounter, from storytelling as a part of clinical ethics.

### Part IV: Psalm: Invitation to Fragmentation

The Cameron story is a fragment, a snapshot moment that captures more about the story of the consultant than about any moral dilemma or ethical analysis and, in fact, more about the consultant's experience of sharing her experience than about particular skills or practices to be evaluated. The "complex range of moral considerations" are available, but kaleidoscopically – in fragments, not yet organized or cohering into a telescopic lens with the long view forward, up and out, or sharpened into the microscopic lens of fine-grained analysis, though both of those are available if one chooses. I'm sharing the encounter as a fragment of a consult – and have shared these fragments of my thinking about it – pulling from and pointing to the different thoughts and ideas that flit and flutter around this experience and my experience of telling it. I've decided to leave this concluding story as inconclusive, incomplete, as an invitation to the reader to look for what is meaningful – what stands out, what they would want to know or have cleared up or where they'd find resources or references for reflection and learning. What sings to them or whispers in these kinds of moments? This story is a story in process to illustrate and model the story *of processing* as part of our responsibility as clinical ethics consultations, in and for clinical ethics consultation.

The Cameron story and subsequent reflections are an example of the messiness of meaning-making in the moral encounters we call our day-jobs. As an example, it is an invitation to the reader – to peers and colleagues and students and trainees – to be explicit and open in sharing your stories in their unfolding and messiness – to invite others to uncover the meanings available in your experience that you didn't know were there. I invite the listener/reader to not get caught by the frames of completion and the comprehensive at the expense of the possibilities for comprehension. I'm leaving this story here – unfinished and raw, troubling and naïve to many of its meanings in the hopes others might do the same with the stories of their experiences. It will for sure make for a messier collection of recollections in the field.[36] Such narratives, such stories will likely reveal the still-present fault lines among our community: the ongoing variations in practices, underlying commitments and understandings of the work of clinical ethics, the goals and aspirations of what professionalization means. Since these fault lines and variations exist anyway, perhaps being more explicit about those will be helpful. Like in a consultation, the deep underlying issues, taken for granted, get raised to the surface in the encounter with the other, with strangers, within strange lands and circumstances. As ethics consultants, we often embody – literally – the opportunity to explore and discover what is actually going on and actually at stake for patients, families, clinicians, and others. Perhaps we can do so with and for each other in sharing *our* stories of *our experiences*, rather than relying on the convention and safety of only turning encounters with patients into cases for analysis.

Perhaps not, and for sure the forces aligned against such openness and professional vulnerability and clinical (and existential) unfinished-ness are many and strong. But just as part of our work entails inviting and listening to and for the voices of those with something at stake in the moral encounter, I would like to believe in (I am oriented toward and committed to valuing) the potential benefit of such storytelling. And I would like to encourage and see us as a field or a cohort of practicing clinical ethicists, invite and listen to and for each others' voices, because like it or not, we are at stake in these conversations as well.

## Notes

1  Wolff, Kurt H. (1976). Surrender and Catch: Experience and Inquiry Today. In *Boston Studies in the Philosophy and History of Science*, vol. 51. Dordrecht: Springer. pp. 29–31.
2  Finder, Stuart G. (2018). The Zadeh Scenario. In Stuart G. Finder and Mark J. Bliton (eds.), *Peer Review, Peer Education, and Modeling in the Practice of Clinical Ethics Consultation: The Zadeh Project*. Cham, Switzerland: Springer Verlag. pp. 21–42. p. 27; Zaner, Richard M. (2010). On the Telling of Stories. In Osborne P. Wiggins and Annette Allen (eds.), *Ethics Histories in Clinical Medicine: Essays in Honor of Richard M Zaner*. Springer. pp. 193–210. pp. 204–205 (hereafter TOS).
3  Birkerts, Sven. (2007). *The Art of Time in Memoir: Then, Again*. Minneapolis, MN: Greywolf. p. 9.
4  Henry, Joe. Interview. *The Drop* at the Grammy Museum, Los Angeles, CA. December 12, 2019.
5  Heinlein, R.A. (1953). *Starman Jones*. New York, NY: Ballantine Books. p. 115.
6  Zaner, Richard M. (2015). *A Critical Examination of Ethics in Health Care and Biomedical Research: Voices and Visions*. Springer. pp. 143–146 (hereafter VAV).
7  Deerfield, Corey. (2018). *The Rabbit Listened*. New York, NY: Random House/Dial Books.
8  Hardwig, J. (1997). Autobiography, Biography, and Narrative Ethics. In H. Lindeman (ed.), *Stories and Their Limits: Narrative Approaches to Bioethics*. New York, NY: Routledge. pp. 50–64.
9  Zaner, VAV, 148.
10  Chambers, Tod S. (2019). Toward the polyphonic case. *Hastings Center Report* 49 (6):10–12.
11  Wolff, 54.
12  Engelhardt, H. Tristam (2013). Courage: Facing and Living with Moral Diversity. Remarks at the reception of the Life-Time Achievement Award from The American Society for Bioethics and Humanities. October 25, 2013.
13  Lopez, Barry (1990). *Crow and Weasel*. San Francisco, CA: North Point Press. p. 48.
14  Wiesel, Elie (1997). *A Beggar in Jerusalem*. New York, NY: Schocken; Reprint edition. p. 4.
15  Zaner, TOS, 204.
16  Bourdieu, Pierre. (1999). Understanding. In Pierre Bourdieu (ed.), *The Weight of the World: Social Suffering in Contemporary Society*. Cambridge, UK: Polity Press. pp. 607–626.
17  Ofstad, Harald (1974). Education versus growth in moral development. *The Monist* 58 (4):581–599; Frolic, Andrea (2011). Who are we when we are doing what we are doing? The case for mindful embodiment in ethics case consultation. *Bioethics* 25 (7):370–382.
18  Chambers, 2019.
19  Lopez, 46–48.
20  Bartlett, Virginia L., Bartlett, Shane K., Bliton, Mark J., and Finder, Stuart G. (2015). *The Oral History of Healthcare Ethics: Volume 1: A Life in Clinical Philosophy: A Conversation with Richard M. Zaner*. Video available: http://ohhe.org
21  Schmich, Mary (1997). Advice, Like Youth, Probably Wasted on the Young, *Chicago Tribune*, June 6 1997.
22  Zaner, VAV, 143.
23  Williams, Dar. (1995). You're Aging Well. *The Honesty Room*. Razor and Tie Productions.
24  Henry, Interview. 12/12/19
25  *Ibid.*
26  Williams, Dar. (1996). Iowa (Travelling III). *Mortal City*. Razor and Tie Productions.
27  Birkerts, 23.

28 Zaner, VAV, 143.
29 Bartlett, Virginia L. and Bliton, Mark J. (2022). Philosophizing still: A brief reintroduction to clinical philosophy. *American Journal of Bioethics* 22 (12):43–46.
30 Zaner, VAV, 142–143.
31 Lorde, Audre. (1979). "Women and Honor: Some Notes on Lying.". First published as a pamphlet by Motheroot Press in 1977 and collected in *On Lies, Secrets, and Silence*, 1979 (WW Norton). Rich first read the "notes" at a women writers' workshop in Oneonta, New York, in 1975.
32 Zaner, Richard M. (2006). The phenomenon of vulnerability in clinical encounters. *Human Studies* 29 (3):283–294.
33 Bliton, Mark J. and Finder, Stuart G. (2018). The Zadeh Project – A Frame for Understanding the Generative Ideas, Formation, and Design. In Stuart G. Finder and Mark J. Bliton (eds.), *Peer Review, Peer Education, and Modeling in the Practice of Clinical Ethics Consultation: The Zadeh Project*. Cham, Switzerland: Springer Verlag. pp. 1–18. Finder, fn 2.
34 Finder, Stuart G. and Bliton, Mark J. (2018). Peer Review and Responsibility in/as/for/to Practice. In Stuart G. Finder & Mark J. Bliton (eds.), *Peer Review, Peer Education, and Modeling in the Practice of Clinical Ethics Consultation: The Zadeh Project*. Cham, Switzerland: Springer Verlag. pp. 207–228; Schutz, Alfred (1962). Some Leading Concepts of Phenomenology. In Maurice Natanson (ed.), *Collected Papers of Alfred Schutz: The Problem of Social Reality*, vol. 1. The Hague: Martinus Nijhoff. pp. 99–206; Schutz, Alfred (1970). *Reflections on the Problem of Relevance*. New Haven, CT: Yale University Press. pp. 23–24.
35 Zaner, TOS, 203.
36 Bartlett, Virginia L., Bliton, Mark J., and Finder, Stuart G. (2016). Just a collection of recollections: Clinical ethics consultation and the interplay of evaluating voices. *HEC Forum* 28 (4):301–320.

## Bibliography

Bartlett, Virginia L., Bartlett, Shane K., Bliton, Mark J., and Finder, Stuart G. (2015). *The Oral History of Healthcare Ethics: Volume 1: A life in Clinical Philosophy: A Conversation with Richard M. Zaner*. Video available: http://ohhe.org
Bartlett, Virginia L., Bliton, Mark J., and Finder, Stuart G. (2016). Just a collection of recollections: Clinical ethics consultation and the interplay of evaluating voices. *HEC Forum* 28 (4):301–320.
Bartlett, Virginia L. and Bliton, Mark J. (2022). Philosophizing still: A brief reintroduction to clinical philosophy. *American Journal of Bioethics* 22 (12):43–46.
Birkerts, Sven (2007). *The Art of Time in Memoir: Then, Again*. Minneapolis, MN: Greywolf Press.
Bliton, Mark J. and Finder, Stuart G. (2018). The Zadeh Project – A Frame for Understanding the Generative Ideas, Formation, and Design. In Stuart G. Finder and Mark J. Bliton (eds.), *Peer Review, Peer Education, and Modeling in the Practice of Clinical Ethics Consultation: The Zadeh Project*. Cham, Switzerland: Springer Verlag. pp. 1–18.
Bourdieu, Pierre (1999). Understanding. In Pierre Bourdieu (ed.), *The Weight of the World: Social Suffering in Contemporary Society*. Cambridge, UK: Polity Press. pp. 607–626.
Chambers, Tod S. (2019). Toward the polyphonic case. *Hastings Center Report* 49 (6):10–12.
Doerrfeld, Cori (2018). *The Rabbit Listened*. New York, NY: Random House/Dial Books.
Engelhardt, H. Tristam. (2013). Courage: Facing and living with moral diversity. Remarks at the Reception of the Life-Time Achievement Award from The American Society for Bioethics and Humanities. October 25, 2013.
Finder, Stuart G. (2018). The Zadeh Scenario. In Stuart G. Finder and Mark J. Bliton (eds.), *Peer Review, Peer Education, and Modeling in the Practice of Clinical Ethics Consultation: The Zadeh Project*. Springer Verlag. pp. 21–42.
Finder, Stuart G. and Bliton, Mark J. (2018). Peer Review and Responsibility in/as/for/to Practice. In Stuart G. Finder and Mark J. Bliton (eds.), *Peer Review, Peer Education, and Modeling in the Practice of Clinical Ethics Consultation: The Zadeh Project*. Springer Verlag. pp. 207–228.
Frolic, Andrea (2011). Who are we when we are doing what we are doing? The case for mindful embodiment in ethics case consultation. *Bioethics* 25 (7):370–382.
Hardwig, J. (1997). Autobiography, Biography, and Narrative Ethics. In H. Lindeman (ed.), *Stories and Their Limits: Narrative Approaches to Bioethics*. New York, NY: Routledge. pp. 50–64.
Henry, Joe (2019). Personal notes from live performance/interview. *The Drop* at the Grammy Museum, Los Angeles, CA. December 12, 2019.

Heinlein, Robert. A. (1953). *Starman Jones*. New York, NY: Ballantine Books.

Lopez, Barry (1990). *Crow and Weasel*. San Francisco, CA: North Point Press. p. 48.

Lorde, Audre. (1979). "Women and Honor: Some Notes on Lying." First published as a pamphlet by Motheroot Press in 1977 and collected in *On Lies, Secrets, and Silence*, 1979 (New York: WW Norton).

Ofstad, Harald (1974). Education versus growth in moral development. *The Monist* 58 (4):581–599.

Rasmussen, Lisa (2018). Standardizing the Case Narrative. In Stuart G. Finder and Mark J. Bliton (eds.), *Peer Review, Peer Education, and Modeling in the Practice of Clinical Ethics Consultation: The Zadeh Project*. Springer Verlag. pp. 151–160.

Schmich, Mary (1997). Advice, Like Youth, Probably Wasted on the Young, *Chicago Tribune*, June 6, 1997.

Schutz, Alfred (1962). Some Leading Concepts of Phenomenology. In Maurice Natanson (ed.), *Collected Papers of Alfred Schutz: The Problem of Social Reality*, vol. 1. The Hague: Martinus Nijhoff. pp. 99–206.

Schutz, Alfred (1970). *Reflections on the Problem of Relevance*. New Haven, CT: Yale University Press. pp. 23–24.

Wiesel, Elie (1997). *A Beggar in Jerusalem*. New York, NY: Schocken; Reprint edition.

Williams, Dar (1995). You're Aging Well. *The Honesty Room*. Razor & Tie Productions.

Williams, Dar (1996). Iowa (Travelling III). *Mortal City*. Razor and Tie Productions.

Wolff, Kurt H. (1976). Surrender and Catch: Experience and Inquiry Today. In *Boston Studies in the Philosophy and History of Science*, vol. 51. Dordrecht: Springer. pp. 29–31.

Zaner, Richard M. (2006). The phenomenon of vulnerability in clinical encounters. *Human Studies* 29 (3):283–294.

Zaner, Richard M. (2010). On the Telling of Stories. In Osborne P Wiggins and Annette Allen (eds.), *Ethics Histories in Clinical Medicine: Essays in Honor of Richard M Zaner*. Springer. pp. 193–210.

Zaner, Richard M. (2015). *A Critical Examination of Ethics in Health Care and Biomedical Research: Voices and Visions*. Springer.

# Sharing Stories with Strangers

## Continuing When There Is No Ending

### Notes on Storytelling – Clinical and Otherwise

The thing about clinical stories is that they can be transformative, illuminating, and educational without being evaluative or evaluated. Stories may not need the bold-typed moral at the end like a fable from Aesop. They don't have to be overtly normative, like Dr Suess's *Wacky Wednesday*, where the reader is expected to spot *what's wrong with this picture*. They don't usually follow the discernable arc of the Hero's Journey. Clinical stories don't offer much if they are framed as straight morality plays, like my toddler's favorite, *Dragons Love Tacos*, where everything goes up in flames because someone's enthusiasm and intention to do something good meant they didn't remember all the warnings to be careful and pay attention to the fine print. But whether clinical stories resemble fables or memoirs, children's stories or histories, we learn from listening and telling about the experiences we share as humans – by communicating in and through our clinical stories.

The practice of sharing stories is thus a clinical practice. Bliton and Finder introduce *The Zadeh Project* by framing clinical ethics work as communicative and acknowledging the expansive range of communications through which clinical ethics consultants work. They write,

> the clinical and moral work of clinical ethics consultation is primarily communicative, involving many varied forms of telling and listening, which thereby elicit additional repetitions, including written forms, to establish clearly, to the extent possible, what is morally relevant.[1]

The aim of clinical storytelling as an element of practice is discovering what is morally relevant, which carries with it serious questions of how to "to express the complex range and scope of moral considerations that are generated as well as evoked through ethics consultation work."[2] As the examples of the *Zadeh Project* and the "Cameron story" in Chapter 6 illustrate, the initial telling or writing may be automatic – a reaction to the weight and movement, the earth-shaking uncertainty of an encounter in a clinical context. Get it out! Write it down! Experiential emesis has its value, after all. But through the method, the discipline of responsible practice, comes the clean-up: the reflection, the reconsiderations, and the examination and engagement with what remains on the page (or hangs in the air if the dialogue is oral and aural). The story itself, the telling, beckons and demands a response: What now? What next? What do I make of this? What do I do with this? *What does this mean? To these others I've encountered? To me?*

That question of meaning itself can seem so heavy and uncertain that much of the writing on clinical ethics focuses on reducing the consultation to something more manageable: a case report, a dueling either/or, point-counterpoint, an analogous situation, paradigms we've pinned down in previous work. Albert Jonsen's "cases are the common coin of medical ethics"[3] has turned into aiming for equal measure in all things: shearing off the bumpy parts and thorny branches, the tangled roots of actual clinical experiences to get to a recognizable and regularized structure – all

DOI: 10.4324/9781003354864-13

things being equal to allow comparison among "reasonable ethics consultants."[4] After all, if we're going to trade cases as sources of insight and meaning, don't we have to agree on what is valuable and how? Narrowing the lens of what gets written, gets reported and gets recognized creates a focus on predetermined issues of a given *kind*, able to be grasped by the widest possible audience in our narrow field of peers – turning the complex meanings of moral encounters into clearly delineated ethical dilemmas, broadly understood if not deeply.

But meanings exceed and escape forms. Meanings rarely behave or follow direction, and they do not stay still or static, even when they pause for a moment's recognition. Which is why we discover and create meaning and meanings in stories – by telling and listening with others – subjecting both the stories and the meanings to "visions and revisions"[5] over time and across contexts. Stories allow for us to "make allowance enough for differences of situation and temper,"[6] to risk and brave understanding another – and understanding ourselves in ways other than we had previously.[7] In clinical encounters, as Zaner points out, we're listening and telling stories with people disrupted, in crisis, thrown into and caught by uncertainty, unchosen and often undesired. We risk doing violence to the concerns and understandings of these others if we start by looking for analogies from *our* conceptual frames, based on *our knowledge* and trying to fit the *sui generis* experience of *these ones involved here and now* into the boxes or paradigms or models we find helpful or "right." We risk missing the potential solutions that might be meaningful for them, in light of their needs and values. Both the ill or injured person, disrupted and caught in an unchosen experience of uncertainty and unknowing, and the care provider wrestling with their own limitations of unknowing and uncertainty, are trying to make sense of and find meaning in their situation and its various options for actions and possible outcomes. In the relationships of patient to care providers and (perhaps) to ethics consultants, presentations of uncertainty and the need-to-know arrive in story form: as descriptions of contexts, experiences, facts as known or under question, hypotheticals and imagined futures, spun together from the threads of other experiences, stories, facts, beliefs, values, imaginings, and hopes. The work of clinical ethics, thus, is listening to and feeling the weight of those threads, helping see connections and weaving together meanings and understandings when possible.

Yet in doing so, the story of *that* work doesn't often get told. We're so busy turning others' stories into cases – to be presented and analyzed or debated or held up as models (or warnings) – that we miss (or outright avoid) the opportunity to share our experiences of finding or making meaning in and through and about the work that we do. As Zaner noted in 2015's *Visions and Voices*:

> Perhaps the most neglected facet of clinical ethics consultation has been the curious failure to appreciate that the ethicist, however understood, does in fact get involved and that involvement has its inevitable consequences on the ethicist him/herself. *I myself am at stake in my clinical involvements, like it or not what happens in these conversations affects me"* (emphasis mine). If others are helped or harmed, so is the ethicist, for the act of involvement is necessarily reflexive, it reverberates back onto the ethicists in distinctive ways quite as much as it has its own kind of effect on the other clinical participants.[8]

The ethics consultant – by their involvement in and attention to the moral encounter – becomes responsible to and for that encounter, including the stories that emerge. Even in responsibility that is shared with others – the ethics consultant's responsibility is elemental to the practice. The clinical ethics consultant is responsible for hearing and holding the cacophony of voices, all desperate to understand and be understood. Listening and telling stories helps discover what makes sense and what may be meaningful, even if the consultation encounter started in uncertainty and confusion.

The experiences of and the meanings such responsibilities carry and create for the ethics consultant are hard to talk about, so we distill the stories of our encounters with patients and healthcare providers into cases for analysis and presentation and we relate them in impersonal, generalized forms.

But it is possible to tell different stories. Zaner, Finder and Bliton, and a few others offer a different form, acknowledging that the specific consultant, a particular *me*, answers the call when listening to the stories of those in need and in their unknowing. Zaner's narrative work, especially as described in the context of vulnerability in Chapter 5, along with *The Zadeh Project*, conceived of and executed by my teachers and colleagues, Finder and Bliton, are examples of engaging with the moral experiences and the practical, actual doing of clinical ethics consultants in their work. This book of mine has emerged from those currents, although this project is different than either Zaner's efforts or *the Zadeh project*. Rather than exploring philosophical concerns with clinical stories or offering multiple perspectives on a single story, I have explored and shared multiple stories in pursuit of a singular and ongoing question: what is it like to do this work and do it responsibly? After swimming through the wide river of influences and ideas that lead to this question and this book, I hope *Sharing Stories with Strangers* will prove as inviting to others in our field as the stories that beckoned to me: Come on in! The water's great!

## Continuing *Because* There Is No Ending

In *Sharing Stories with Strangers,* each chapter, each story, highlights and focuses on a particular element of the clinical ethicist's responsibility. The focus on each element emerged over time with reflection on the particular circumstances, the stories generated and through the various philosophical, clinical, literary, or artistic resources that illuminate the experience and the element at hand. Each chapter is a weaving-together of both the experience and what I have found helpful in thinking through such experiences, trying to engage what Finder and Bliton describe as a "primary task … of finding the best way and to employ in the most faithful way to express the complex range and scope of moral considerations."[9]

The stories in this collection are personal and particular – experienced, written and reflected on throughout my clinical ethics education, training, and practice. They have been shared and collected over the past several years, and I have struggled to bring them together to tell a story about clinical ethics work, to present a narrative that might resonate with others in the field, might serve as access and invitation to those entering the field. It never quite worked, and it wasn't until the COVID-19 pandemic brought so much into question – personally, professionally, publicly, politically that the questions about practice that prompted writing this book became clearer in important ways. Amid the clamor of public and institutional demands for Bioethics answers, the questions emerged (again) of what responsibility means in clinical ethics practice. I realized that in my efforts "to get the story right,"[10] I'd almost overlooked that it is *the practice* of telling the *multiple* and *varied* stories about how we do what we do in our work that matters: the experience of listening and telling, together.

So, instead of building a singular story from these many pieces, I have gathered them and sat with them, walked through them again and again, rewritten them and retold them to myself and to others: trying to discover what threads of connection and meaning run through the stories – individually and together. I have revisited philosophers and poets and clinicians, researchers and teachers, artists and musicians –even the authors of children's books that speak to different registers of experience – to learn again how others make sense of the moral encounters described in their writings, songs, and stories, to discover what I might learn from their experiences as I continue to learn through mine.

What has emerged is *Sharing Stories with Strangers,* this collection of recollections, a series of clinical stories, and the reflections they have generated at the time of the encounters, and over time since. They invite question and response, listening and telling, emerging as they did from personal experiences and a deep tradition of ethics consultants as phenomenologically oriented clinicians:

"hunter/gatherers, seekers and collectors of the stories that make up every clinical encounter … listening to and learning to understand such stories also witnesses and guarantees, ensuring that every clinical narrative has its chance to be told and receives its appropriate hearing."[11]

I wrote this book to focus attention on clinical ethics consultants' experiences which have not, historically, gotten their appropriate hearing. My hope is sharing these stories will provide access and insight into what this work of clinical ethics can be like, and that the book models how we might try to share our stories with each other.

After all, the decades-long gap or absence (or sheer avoidance) of sharing consultants' experiences – perhaps sped up by the move toward professionalization and the ongoing calls for consensus, standardization, and certification – challenges us as individuals trying to practice responsibly, and as members of a field, especially one trying to grow into a profession. As the stories and reflections throughout reveal: your procedures will not protect you. Your good intentions will not redeem you. Your expertise is no match for the "wild serendipity" of the universe[12] and wild uncertainty of human experiences. The moral moment will not be televised.

We learn *continuously* through the stories we tell of our clinical experiences, and the elements and methods of practice they reveal. The discipline of questions. An openness to disruption and an orientation to discovery – paying attention to the facts of our disruption and the how of our paying attention. The weight of recognizing responsibility and the humility of being never quite easy again. The deliberate engagement with our own self-reflection and self-education, bringing each other into our experiences and learning. Practicing, cultivating a curiosity – a wonderment – about the other people we encounter in their specificity and uniqueness: "an understanding – at once unique and general – of each life story."[13] We recognize that our experiences – like those of the other stakeholders in any encounter, create unique vulnerabilities which generate stories for making sense of our upheaval and uncertainty. We acknowledge that stories carry responsibilities – to and for each other. As we walk into the stories of others, by invitation or accident, we take them on as parts of our stories – and we are responsible for our role in theirs. Especially those that we write down and send out into the world.

The responsibility for those accumulated stories requires that we share them *as they become part of ours.* Zaner echoes this point noting that writing requires engagement with others: "conversations and writings need to be continually submitted to others for their understandings, but also for their critiques. Understood in this way, writing may be one aspect of a more general method."[14] We write so that we can offer our stories to each other to probe, clarify, co-create, and help bear as witnesses, as Bourdieu writes, helping to "create the conditions for an extraordinary discourse, which might never have been spoken, which were already there, merely awaiting the conditions of its actualization."[15] *Sharing Stories with Strangers* highlights our stories as clinical ethics consultants, modeling the elements of responsibility and method the practice requires for understanding together: the orientations and the recognitions that we are each large, that we contain multitudes, and that with space and time and attention, we each can voice what all matters, and how and why, in these extraordinary conversations. After all, as Joe Henry once explained about writing a song, "The whole process is deeply and unfailingly personal … but it's subject is not." In sharing the personal, particular clinical ethics stories we stumble through "the various tellings and yellings" which, like clinical ethics encounters themselves, in the end, "are efforts – some still tentative, some more vigorous – to make sense of things and in the end, of ourselves, of our lives."[16] In that sharing, and with a promise to hear each other's stories in whatever forms they emerge, we create the possibility of understanding and learning, together, about the interpersonal, shared experiences that shape our practices of clinical ethics consultation.

## Notes

1 Bliton, Mark J. and Finder, Stuart G. (2018). The Zadeh Project – A Frame for Understanding the Generative Ideas, Formation, and Design. In Stuart G. Finder and Mark J. Bliton (eds.), Peer Review, Peer Education, and Modeling in the Practice of Clinical Ethics Consultation: The Zadeh Project. Springer Verlag. p. 2.
2 *Ibid.* 5.
3 Jonsen, Albert R. (1991). Casuistry as methodology in clinical ethics. *Theoretical Medicine* 12 (4):295–307.

4 Rasmussen, Lisa (2018). Standardizing the Case Narrative. In Stuart G. Finder and Mark J. Bliton (eds.), Peer Review, Peer Education, and Modeling in the Practice of Clinical Ethics Consultation: The Zadeh Project. Springer Verlag. pp. 151–160.

5 Eliot, T.S. (1915) *The Love Song of J. Alfred Prufrock.* https://poets.org/poem/love-song-j-alfred-prufrock

6 Austen, Jane. (1813). Pride and Prejudice. New York: Signet Classic edition 1989. p. 117.

7 Wolff, Kurt H. (1976). Surrender and Catch: Experience and Inquiry Today. In *Boston Studies in the Philosophy and History of Science*, vol. 51. Dordrecht: Springer. p. 24.

8 Zaner, Richard M. (2015). *A Critical Examination of Ethics in Health Care and Biomedical Research: Voices and Visions.* Dordrecht: Springer. p. 148.

9 Bliton and Finder, 5.

10 Zaner, Richard M. (2010). On the Telling of Stories. In Osborne P. Wiggins and Annette Allen (eds.), *Ethics Histories in Clinical Medicine: Essays in Honor of Richard M. Zaner.* Dordrecht: Springer. pp. 193–210. p. 207.

11 *Ibid.*

12 "I have been met by the universe with wild serendipity." Joe Henry, with Grayson Haver Currin, "Joe Henry's Next Second Chance" *National Public Radio* interview. November 15, 2019. https://www.npr.org/2019/11/15/779415463/joe-henry-album-gospel-according-to-water-cancer-second-chance

13 Bourdieu, Pierre (1999). Understanding. In Pierre Bourdieu (ed.), *The Weight of the World: Social Suffering in Contemporary Society.* Cambridge, UK: Polity Press. pp. 607–626, p. 614.

14 Zaner, 207.

15 Bourdieu, 614.

16 Zaner, 207.

## Bibliography

Austen, Jane. (1813) Pride and Prejudice. New York: Signet Classic edition 1989.

Bliton, Mark J. and Finder, Stuart G. (2018). The Zadeh Project – A Frame for Understanding the Generative Ideas, Formation, and Design. In Stuart G. Finder and Mark J. Bliton (eds.), *Peer Review, Peer Education, and Modeling in the Practice of Clinical Ethics Consultation: The Zadeh Project.* Cham, Switzerland: Springer Verlag.

Bourdieu (1999). Understanding. In Pierre Bourdieu (eds.), *The Weight of the World: Social Suffering in Contemporary Society.* Cambridge, UK: Polity Press. pp. 607–626.

Eliot, T.S. (1915) *The Love Song of J. Alfred Prufrock.* https://poets.org/poem/love-song-j-alfred-prufrock

Henry, Joe and Currin, Grayson Haver (2019). Joe Henry's next second chance. *National Public Radio* interview. November 15, 2019. https://www.npr.org/2019/11/15/779415463/joe-henry-album-gospel-according-to-water-cancer-second-chance

Jonsen, Albert R. (1991). Casuistry as methodology in clinical ethics. *Theoretical Medicine* 12 (4):295–307.

Rasmussen, Lisa (2018). Standardizing the Case Narrative. In Stuart G. Finder and Mark J. Bliton (eds.), *Peer Review, Peer Education, and Modeling in the Practice of Clinical Ethics Consultation: The Zadeh Project.* Cham, Switzerland: Springer Verlag. pp. 151–160.

Wolff, Kurt H. (1976). Surrender and Catch: Experience and Inquiry Today. In *Boston Studies in the Philosophy and History of Science*, vol. 51. Dordrecht: Springer.

Zaner, Richard M. (2010). On the Telling of Stories. In Osborne P. Wiggins and Annette Allen (eds.), *Ethics Histories in Clinical Medicine: Essays in Honor of Richard M Zaner.* Cham, Switzerland: Springer. pp. 193–210.

Zaner, Richard M. (2015). *A Critical Examination of Ethics in Health Care and Biomedical Research: Voices and Visions.* Dordrecht: Springer.

# Index

Note: Page references with "n" denote endnotes.

For Product Safety Concerns and Information please contact our
EU representative GPSR@taylorandfrancis.com Taylor & Francis
Verlag GmbH, Kaufingerstraße 24, 80331 München, Germany